S0-BAT-270

The Practical Art
of Medicine

The Practical Art of Medicine

Robert B. Taylor, M. D.

Medical Department
Harper & Row Publishers, Inc.
Hagerstown, Maryland
New York, Evanston, San Francisco, London

The Practical Art of Medicine. Copyright © 1972 by
Harper & Row, Publishers, Inc. All rights reserved. No part
of this book may be used or reproduced in any manner
whatsoever without written permission except in the case
of brief quotations embodied in critical articles and reviews.
Printed in The United States of America. For information
address Medical Department, Harper & Row, Publishers,
Inc., 2350 Virginia Avenue, Hagerstown, Maryland 21740.

Standard Book Number: 06–142543–5

Library of Congress Catalog Card Number: 72–83808

. . . To a physician of another generation

When I began collecting notes for this book, a colleague suggested that I write to his old preceptor—a small-town New England family physician who had served his patients and guided the destinies of medical students for decades. "He knows more practical medicine than any man I ever met. Once he spent an hour teaching me how to bandage a finger properly. Over and over we practiced, until I finally had it right."

My letter was never answered. The doctor had died the week before.

"What a loss, that all his knowledge should die with him," I said.

My friend smiled. "His knowledge didn't die with him."

I knew what he meant.

To this devoted physician and the thousands like him who over the years made the house calls, offered hope when medicine failed, fought disease with ingenuity when equipment was lacking, yet found time to pass their knowledge to the new generation of physicians, THE PRAC-TICAL ART OF MEDICINE is dedicated.

Contents

Preface

The practice of medicine is a very personal art—an intense meeting of the minds to solve a physical or emotional problem. Generations of physicians have refined the format of the diagnostic interview and our libraries are filled with a wealth of medical knowledge, but in solving day-to-day clinical problems, the practicing physician must often deal innovatively with diagnostic puzzles and unusual injuries.

American medical practice today is a "cottage" industry. Whether the doctor's cottage is a medical center office or a quiet building in the country, as is mine, each of us evolves practical solutions to everyday medical problems. By picking the brains of colleagues, scanning the literature, and using "yankee ingenuity," the physician develops his individual style. He learns to examine shy infants without evoking tears, to remove a kaleidoscopic array of foreign bodies from orifices, to repair unlikely injuries, and to resist intimidation by third parties. Somehow the physician must learn to maintain useful, legible records, charge and collect fair fees for his services, and squeeze into each busy day a little time for relaxation.

For these problems, I have found the techniques and tips described in THE PRACTICAL ART OF MEDICINE to be the most efficient solutions. Some come from books and journals, others from older and wiser physicians, some from my nursing staff, and a few from give-and-take with patients.

If even a single tip helps solve a diagnostic problem, prevents suffering and grief, or gives a physician an extra hour to spend with his family, then the effort has been worthwhile.

Acknowledgments

No book is a solo venture, and many persons contributed to the preparation of this volume. I wish to acknowledge the long hours of manuscript typing by Carol Ostmark, assisted by Patricia McCann, Helen Roberts, and Mary Ellen Rebhan. I thank Dorothy Dolce, Medical Librarian of the Kingston City Hospital, Kingston, New York, for her assistance in providing reference material, and Elizabeth Graff for preparing many of the illustrations.

The persons who offered specific tips and afforded consultation are too many to list, but I wish to express my sincere appreciation for their contributions. Certain procedures and tips have previously appeared in print in *Medical Economics, Physician's Management, Private Practice, Emergency Medicine,* and *Resident and Staff Physician;* they are reprinted here with the permission of the publishers.

I extend a special thank-you to my most photogenic patients—Sharon Taylor, Diana Taylor, Mr. and Mrs. O.C. Taylor, and my wife Anita.

The Practical Art
of Medicine

Introduction:
What You Didn't Learn in Medical School

What you didn't learn in medical school fills volumes: This is one of them!

Our heritage of medical knowledge passes from one generation to the next, both within and outside the medical school walls. Modern medical education has its roots in the master-student-apprentice relation that dates back to the time of Hippocrates. Over the centuries, innovative clinicians have devised practical solutions to vexing problems, enriching the legacy of medical knowledge passed to the new physician.

In 1819, René Laennec used a cylinder to listen to his patient's chest instead of following his predecessors' intimate but awkward method of placing the ear directly on the chest wall. A simple innovation, at first utilizing only a rolled-up sheet of paper, later refined into the monaural stethoscope, this practical device earned for Laennec a place among the great clinicians of the ages.

The superabundance of medical knowledge available today makes the education of a physician long and arduous. Medical school has been described as an endurance test rather than an educational experience. Certainly, every physician must be familiar with kwashiorkor and the Hand-Schüller-Christian syndrome, even though he will probably never see a patient with either disease. He must have at least a passing knowledge of yaws, scurvy, silo-filler's disease, the Taussig-Bing syndrome, heart transplants, and the Australia antigen.

It takes time to drum all this information into the student's cranium. In the last century, Henry McMurtrie recognized the proliferation of medical knowledge and the years that must be devoted to its acquisition: "Boys, don't study medicine. By the time you earn your bread, you will have no teeth left to eat it with."

During the years of studying obscure conditions, there is little time available for learning trivia—minor details, such as how to get an angry bug out of the patient's ear, how to get a ring off a swollen finger without a ring cutter, how to do a pelvic examination on a bedfast patient, how to remove a Foley catheter when the balloon won't deflate, how to find a vein in the patient who seems to have none, how to schedule patients to avoid a jam in the waiting room, how to persuade the patient who demands a house call that he really wants to come into the office, how to train an aide, how to recognize when practice expenses are too high, and how to get home in time for dinner.

When I left medical school 10 years ago, my classmates and I were presented with diplomas asserting our proficiency to practice medicine and surgery, and cast adrift like ships without rudders, floundering at the mercy of third parties, federal agencies, office equipment salesmen, bank managers, tax investigators, and of course, patients. We had no real instruction in how to make a living at the craft we had been taught.

Times are changing, but slowly. Medical schools now devote a few hours to the consideration of medical economics, grudgingly admitting that their white-coated protégés will soon be treating real live private patients and will soil their hands with dollars.

The Practical Art of Medicine records the treatment methods and office procedures of our generation of clinicians. In this book, you will find helpful tips that may, like Laennec's stethoscope, be standard medical practice during the next decade. I shall discuss office administration and collection methods, offer hints on how to avoid being bullied by insurance companies, lawyers, and government agencies, and pass along some clues to finding happiness in your day-by-day medical practice.

The Practical Art of Medicine presents the utilitarian clinical methods of medical practice today, together with hundreds of useful tips to save you time, effort, grief, and money. The longer you have been in practice, the more familiar you will be with the topics in this book.

Each generation of physicians passes the torch to the next, along with the ever-growing treasury of modern medical knowledge. For the new generation of physicians—with untempered knowledge, untarnished ethics, and unbounded hope for the future of medicine in America— *The Practical Art of Medicine* is written.

1

The Mysteries of Diagnosis

There is no royal road to diagnosis.

Robert Tuttle Morse
(1857–1945)

The medical consultation is rigidly structured, the end result of centuries of trial and error by physicians. The rules have been laid down. Ignore them at your peril!

The patient in your office understands (perhaps instinctively) what constitutes the thorough evaluation of his problem. He'll sense any shortcut and wonder why. Be fair to the patient and yourself; follow the rules, and you will be rewarded by the confidence of your patients and a high batting average in diagnosis.

Good medical practice dictates, and the patient expects, a thorough medical history followed by a physical examination of all areas in question. Next comes the diagnosis, the physician's assertion that he understands what is wrong. Treatment follows the diagnosis and may range from simple reassurance to a complicated regimen of therapy.

Sounds elementary, doesn't it? But haven't you some time recently skirted one of those steps, cutting the history short or abbreviating the physical examination, only to suffer later embarrassment or worse?

THE DIAGNOSTIC INTERVIEW

The diagnostic interview is a brief but intense meeting of minds. It must be more than filling in the blanks on a history form; that can be done by computer. The interview can't be conducted over the telephone, and it can't be handled by the office nurse. You must sit with the patient, look him in the eye, put your pen aside, and find out what is wrong!

Why is the patient in the office today? What is he worried about? Is he really discussing the problem that prompted him to call for an appointment? What does he want from the doctor?

Anxiety brings most patients to the doctor's office. In the tenth century Ali ibn-Hazm wrote: "No one is moved to act, or resolves to speak a single word, who does not hope by means of this action or word to release anxiety from his spirit." The patient visits the doctor because he is worried about a problem. There is usually some fantasy about the disease. The patient with a harmless external hemorrhoid is worried about cancer; the housewife with aching joints has heard of a friend's aunt who was crippled by arthritis. Find out exactly what the patient is worried about and deal with his anxieties; if you don't, his visit will be a failure.

Watch your patient! What is he really saying? Watch his eyes and hands. Do they become restless when he discusses one aspect of the complaint? Recognize the nonverbal clues.

Sometimes the complaint seems trivial—a headache or mild indigestion. Find out how your patient feels about his problem. "What do you think might be wrong?" "What brings you in *today?*" "Is there anything special about this problem that has been worrying you?" Ask yourself, "Why is this patient here today?"

Try to elicit information by inference rather than direct questioning. Don't assault your patient with an emotionally charged interrogation. In *Diseases of the Heart and Circulation,* Paul Hamilton Wood wrote: "The best history taker is he who can best interpret the answer to a leading question."

"Tell me about it." "Can you think of anything that might be causing your headache or indigestion?" "Is there anything else you should tell me?"

Use all your clues. Did a workman lose a day's work to see you today? Why? The patient with a seemingly stable condition calls at 3 A.M. Why? Does the patient mention something only to assure you it has nothing to do with his problem? Why? Wilfred Trotter (1872–1939) wrote: "Disease often tells its secrets in a casual parenthesis." Minutia, trivia, and misstatement can unlock the mysteries of diagnosis.

THE PATIENT'S HISTORY

The **chief complaint** is the reason the patient gives for his visit to the doctor. How long has he had it? How did it begin? Has it changed? Has he had it before? What was the diagnosis then? How was it treated then? How does the patient feel about his symptoms?

How bad is the pain? Often a hard question to answer. Try asking your patient about the worst pain he ever had. "Okay, that is one dollar's worth of pain. Now how much is your present pain worth— twenty-five cents, fifty cents, seventy-five cents?"

What makes the symptoms better? What makes them worse? Are they influenced by eating, drinking, anxiety, exasperation, exercise, rest?

Has the patient done anything about the symptoms? Has he seen another doctor? Has he tried any medication? If so, how did it work? Avoid the embarrassment of writing a prescription for penicillin for a throat infection only to have the patient inform you he has been taking that antibiotic for the past 5 days.

The past medical history should be available in all cases and is often the key to diagnosis. A list of past medical history highlights should appear on the face sheet of your office records, kept up to date, handy for ready reference at each office visit. (This will be discussed in Chapter 19.) Did the patient suffer repeated childhood sore throats? Did he have rheumatic fever? Did he miss several months of school because of illness? Did the doctor restrict any childhood activities? Was he ever rejected for military service, for an insurance policy, or for employment because of health? Did he have a tonsillectomy, adenoidectomy, appendectomy, hernia repair, or severe injury? Was he ever hospitalized? When? Why? Have we forgotten anything?

The occupational history offers important clues in medicine, surgery, and orthopedics. Is your patient a laborer, executive, or housewife? Does he hold two jobs? Has there been a change recently? A promotion? New responsibility? What does he do in his work? Are there repetitive motions that may strain muscles? I care for a number of middle-aged (and older) women who do piecework at local garment mills, spending long hours working hurriedly, crouched over a sewing machine. Over the past few years, every one of them has mentioned having pain in the upper back and shoulders.

Has your patient changed jobs frequently? Did he quit? Was he fired? Why? Has he suffered repeated occupational injuries? Has he had to change employment because of health?

What does the housewife patient do during the day? Does she carry around a 20-lb. baby. Does she tug on a pulley clothesline and wonder why her shoulder hurts? Does she have a hobby?

Habits cause a host of medical problems. Does your patient smoke? Cigar, pipe, cigarette? Does he smoke three cigarettes or three packs? Does he take alcohol? "If you had a fifth of whisky, how long would it last?" Does he drink coffee or tea? How many cups a day? Does he sleep well? What time does he go to bed? What time does he get up?

Allergies can complicate many problems. Is the patient allergic to any medication? Foods? Animals? Watch the patient with an allergy to molds; he may have a violent penicillin reaction. Don't give chick-embryo-derived flu vaccine to patients allergic to chicken or egg.

The family history is a treasury of information. Your patient is the current episode of his family history. Read the past editions to understand the present. A multitude of diseases show familial patterns. Are any diseases common in his family? Did his father or mother have any illnesses? At what age did the illnesses begin? Are his parents alive? Or at what age did they die? What was the cause of death? Do his brothers or sisters have any illnesses? How about his more distant relatives? Is there anything we have forgotten?

Yes, the diagnostic interview takes time. But diagnosis is a puzzle and you need all the pieces. The intern who summarizes the past medical history, social history, and family history with the word "noncontributory" really means that he did not contribute his time to this important diagnostic procedure.

PHYSICAL EXAMINATION

Sir Dominic John Corrigan (1802–1880) wrote: "The trouble with doctors is not that they don't know enough, but that they don't see enough." Your best tools, your five senses, are always with you. The physical examination begins the minute you lay eyes on the patient. Stay alert. How does he walk, talk, behave? Does the patient who complains of a painful shoulder strip off his shirt like a healthy young athlete? Does the patient with a pilonidal cyst stand or sit during the interview?

Follow the rules. Do a thorough physical examination. The patient could have told you his symptoms over the telephone. He came to your office for an examination. Don't cheat him and yourself!

Have the patient remove his clothes. You can't listen to his heart through his shirt. Provide cotton or paper gowns. When you examine a female patient, have a nurse in the room. Be considerate of budding 11-year-old girls; gown them too.

Touch, listen, observe, smell, and taste if necessary. Stand back and take a good look at the whole patient. Determine the blood pressure, pulse, and respiratory rate. Then look in every orifice. Check the ocular fundus. Do tonometry when necessary. Remove dentures and thoroughly inspect the mouth. Don't hesitate to palpate oral lesions. View the tympanic membranes. Palpate the cervical nodes, the supra-clavicular area, the thyroid gland. Feel the thyroid as the patient swallows.

Carefully examine the lungs and heart, following the time-honored ritual of inspection, palpation, percussion, and auscultation. Your stethoscope is as valuable as the best electrocardiograph. It is an extention of your ears, and the sounds you hear through it should be as familiar as your children's voices. Warm that arctic stethoscope head in the palm of your hand before applying it to the patient's warm chest.

The abdomen should also be inspected, palpated, percussed, and auscultated. Learn to percuss an enlarged liver and recognize the tinkling bowel sounds of intestinal obstruction.

Examine the genitalia. Check for hernias. Examine the scrotal contents. Don't neglect the pelvic examination and the all-important Papanicolaou smear.

The thorough physical examination involves a soiled physician's finger. A wag once said he could always tell a specialist; the specialist was the one who did the rectal examination.

Look at the extremities. Feel the pulses. Look at the hair distribution. Are the feet warm or cold?

Don't neglect the neurologic examination. Do sluggish reflexes suggest a thyroid deficiency? How about the patient's vibratory sense? Can he detect a pinprick in the foot?

Make a note about the patient's skin. Is there seborrhea? Are there spider nevi? Pallor? Jaundice?

Have you forgotten anything? Have you recorded the patient's blood pressure while he was relaxed? Have you noted any unusual affect? Posture? Gait? Anything else?

Write it down. The minutes spent in recording a history and physical examination are a small fraction of the time spent in obtaining the data. Don't skimp here. Record negative as well as positive findings; they may be of paramount importance later.

LABORATORY TESTS

Are laboratory tests required in the evaluation of the patient's problem? Don't try to save time here. And don't try to save the patient a little money. The patient has come to you for a thorough evaluation of his problem. If a test is indicated, order it.

Urine analysis is easily performed in the office and should be considered part of every thorough physical examination. Dip-sticks rapidly determine pH and detect protein, glucose, bile, ketones, and blood. Even if the urine is not centrifuged, look at a specimen under the microscope.

Blood Tests can yield valuable information and are necessary to confirm many diagnoses, including diabetes, hepatitis, and anemia.

Electrocardiography is indicated in almost all patients with chest pain and is necessary to differentiate arrhythymias.

X-rays are essential in the diagnosis of many illnesses and injuries. The evaluation of hemoptysis is incomplete without a chest x-ray, and few patients who have suffered trauma should escape without roentgenography.

Other tests that should not be forgotten include examination of the feces, throat culture, sputum examination, and oscillometry.

Now you have taken a careful history, performed a thorough physical examination, and assembled your laboratory reports. The next step is the diagnosis.

DIAGNOSIS

The patient came to you to find out the diagnosis. Don't neglect to tell him. During the first half of the consultation—the history and physical examination—it was the patient's turn to speak. Now it is your turn. What do you think he has?

Tell the patient a diagnosis. You may be able to give him a definitive etiologic diagnosis such as streptococcal pharyngitis or acute myocardial infarction. Or perhaps you must be vague, and your best diagnosis is viral infection or hardening of the arteries. Whatever you do, give him something to report to the family who is anxiously awaiting word from the doctor.

Deal with the patient's fantasies and specifically reassure him about what he does *not* have. "No, that infected hair follicle under your arm is not cancer." "Your headache is due to nervous tension and there is no evidence of an impending stroke."

Diagnose rare conditions only on certain identification. The most common diseases occur most commonly. For every case of lupus erythematosus seen in your practice, there will be 10,000 cases of viral influenza. When you hear hoofbeats, don't look for zebras.

Once you have named the patient's disease, tell him a little about it. Where does the disease come from? Is it contagious? How long will it last? Might the condition recur?

You don't have to tell the patient everything you know about his disease. Don't dazzle him with your brilliant exposition of possible complications, and don't frighten him by describing that case report you read last week. Tell him what he needs to know. Emphasize the important facts. Then outline a course of therapy.

TREATMENT

The patient expects a diagnosis and a course of therapy. If no specific treatment is indicated, reassurance should be provided. Perhaps this is all the patient came for in the first place.

If indicated, a specific regimen of medical or surgical therapy should be outlined. Is medication needed? What is the dose? Will it interfere with other medicine the patient is taking? How long should the medication be taken? Is surgery indicated? Should he see a specialist?

Don't forget the value of nonspecific therapy. Are fluids indicated? Fruit juice? Should the patient take aspirin? How about extra rest? Should he go to school or work? How long should he stay in bed?

What if the treatment doesn't work? Should he call? Should he return for reexamination? Are further tests necessary? Should the patient be referred to a specialist? Don't let the patient out of your office without a specific recommendation concerning what to do if he does not get well.

Keep your treatment simple. A handful of prescriptions brightens the pharmacist's day but confuses the patient. Most common conditions can be treated with one or two simple medications supplemented by general advice concerning diet and rest.

Let's face it! Most of your patients will recover spontaneously if you do nothing. Most medication merely speeds the body's healing process. Samuel J. Meltzer (1851–1920) wrote: "The fact that your patient gets well does not prove that your diagnosis was correct."

Avoid overtreatment. Don't bombard a self-limited viral pharyngitis with penicillin and leave your patient with moniliasis. Watch out for the family doctor–specialist syndrome: The patient visits his family physician repeatedly, describing a new complaint on each visit, and each time adds another medication to his daily quota. Finally, he finds his way to a specialist who, in a bold therapeutic stroke, discontinues all medication, and the patient gets well.

Keep track of your patient. Schedule a revisit when necessary. A telephone call to check on progress takes only a few seconds. Encourage the family to call you if the condition changes. Make yourself available, and you won't find your patient running over to Dr. Jones across town when his stomach pain gets worse.

Finally, in therapy, convince the patient that you are interested. Look him in the eye. Express your concern. And dispense your advice with confidence.

Now the consultation is complete. You have taken a careful history, performed the necessary physical examination, and obtained the indicated laboratory tests. A diagnosis has been made and a course of treatment outlined. The patient has been assured of your interest and cautioned to call if things do not go as expected. For emphasis, repeat the few facts the patient should remember from the interview, stand up, open the door for him, and go on to the next patient.

References and Suggestions for Further Reading

1. Browne K, Freeling P: The Doctor-Patient Relationship. Baltimore, Williams & Wilkins, 1967.
2. Conn H F, Conn R B Jr: Current Diagnosis. Philadelphia, Saunders, 1971.
3. Douthwaite A H: French's Index of Differential Diagnosis. Baltimore, Williams & Wilkins, 1967.
4. Engle R L, Davis B J: Medical diagnosis: Past, present and future: Present concepts of the meaning and limitations of medical diagnosis. Arch Intern Med 112:512–519, 1963.
5. Feinstein A R: Clinical Judgment. Baltimore, Williams & Wilkins, 1967.
6. Feinstein A R, Niebyl J R: Changes in the diagnostic process during 40 years of clinicopathologic conferences. Arch Intern Med 128:774–780, 1971.
7. Harvey A M, Bordley J: Differential Diagnosis: The Interpretation of Clinical Evidence. Philadelphia, Saunders, 1970.
8. Lusted L B: Introduction to Medical Decision Making. Springfield, Ill, Thomas, 1968.
9. MacBryde C M, Blacklow R S: Signs and Symptoms, 5th ed. Philadelphia, Lippincott, 1970.
10. Simborg D W: Experimentation in medical history-taking. JAMA 210:1443–1445, 1969.
11. Stevenson I: The Diagnostic Interview. New York, Harper & Row, 1971.

2
Painless Pediatrics

Children are not simply micro-adults, but have their own specific problems.

Béla Schick
(1877–1967)

Consider the paradox of the pediatrician—a trained and certified specialist—mired in trivia and too rushed to do justice to the referred consultation, all because the slick, ladies' magazines insist the healthy child needs a pediatrician.

Family physicians, answer the call! Lift from the shoulders of your pediatric colleagues the yoke of tedium. Polish your pediatric techniques and encourage your young families to entrust their offspring to your care.

THE WELL BABY CHECK-UPS

The doctor who cares for children spends his day examining well babies and relieving the anxieties of mothers. Beginning with neonatal care in the hospital, the healthy infant visits the doctor every month or two during the first year of life, and the physician should anticipate problems that arise at each stage of the baby's development.

To the new mother, the squalling infant is an unknown entity; she hopes he's normal but is not quite sure. The mother needs to be told at each interview that her healthy baby is growing and developing normally and that she is doing everything right.

The topics for discussion at each visit parallel the baby's development.

The **newborn infant** creates the most maternal anxiety. Spend time with your new mothers. Encourage questions and answer them patiently.

What do new mothers worry about? Neonatal weight loss is normal, up to 10 percent of the birth weight, reaching a maximum at about the third day, followed by a gradual gain in weight. Breast-fed babies lose more weight than bottle-fed babies because, before the "milk comes in" on about the third day, they have to subsist on the scanty amount of colostrum produced. Following the third day of life, breast-fed babies rapidly catch up with their bottle-fed peers.

Is there a jaundiced baby in the nursery? Reassure your mother that jaundice of the newborn is caused by a blood incompatability between mother and baby, and is *not contagious.*

The normal neonatal infant has up to six bowel movements a day, more frequent and softer in breast-fed than in bottle-fed babies; this is normal—not diarrhea, as the anxious new mother may fear.

Breast hypertrophy and "witch's milk" is normal in newborn infants of both sexes.

The umbilical stump will drop off about the fifth day; when it does, the mother should apply alcohol with a cotton-tipped applicator at each diaper change until the site is dry. Then leave the navel alone.

The **2-week check-up** brings mommy and daddy and their new baby for his first office visit. Length and weight measurements are compared with the hospital values. Question the mother concerning nursing or bottle feeding, and ask the mother who is bottle feeding how many ounces the child takes in 24 hours. Examine the infant completely, with careful attention to the skin (jaundice and birthmarks may first be noticed at this time), heart (the murmur of congenital heart disease may not appear until the first week or two of life), navel (check the umbilical stump), and extremities (examine the hips and look for tibial torsion). If the navel is well healed, tell the mother she may begin to tub bathe the baby with a *small* amount of water. Suggest a plastic tub rather than a top-heavy bathinet. (When the baby outgrows the plastic tub, it can be used for soaking clothes.)

Many young mothers come to the 2-week visit complaining, "The baby's formula should be changed. It's not satisfying him." The real cause, of course, is hunger. Junior needs solid food. Begin this 2-week-old infant on cereal feedings, and the crying will stop.

The **6-week check-up** should bring a more confident mother to the office. By now the infant should be taking most cereals and perhaps a few fruits and vegetables. A social smile should be present; be wary of those unsmiling 6-week-old babies. At this visit, the baby begins his routine immunizations with the diphtheria-pertussis-tetanus (DPT) and Sabin oral polio vaccines.

The **10-week check-up** often begins with the question, "Is my baby teething? He chews his gums and drools." No, he's not teething, but is showing the normal increase in saliva at this age. By this time, the infant should be taking all cereals, vegetables, and fruits. The big eater may now begin meat dinners. Some time following 3 months of age, the mother may stop sterilizing and change the formula to homogenized cow's milk or Similac Advance. The 10-week check-up ends with a DPT injection.

By the **3 1/2-month check-up** junior may be able to roll over. He should be eating meat dinners and may be ready to try the more pungent pure meat products. The mother should no longer be sterilizing. The 3½-month visit includes the third DPT and the second dose of oral polio vaccine.

By the **6-month check-up** the baby may really be teething, noisily proclaiming the eruption of each new incisor. He should be able to roll over both ways and may be able to sit without support. Once he has a few teeth, junior foods are begun. Mr. 6-months-old receives his third dose of the Sabin oral polio vaccine.

The **9-month check-up** brings an active infant who can sit, transfer objects from hand to hand, stand with support, and perhaps crawl or walk. By now he has enough teeth to begin soft table food. The 9-month-old infant receives a Tuberculin Tine Test.

By the **1-year check-up** the child should walk, eat table food, and know about three words (mama, dada, and no-no). He should tip the scales at triple his birth weight, a formidable gain. The schedule calls for immunization against rubella, mumps, and measles.

An **annual check-up** is recommended until junior leaves for college. At each visit, the physician should assess the height, weight, motor development, word skills, and general physical condition of the child. Routine immunizations are kept up to date with DPT and Sabin oral polio boosters at ages 2, 5, and 10. The Tuberculin Tine Test should be repeated at 2- to 5-year intervals, varying with the possibility of tuberculosis exposure in the community.

THE PEDIATRIC HISTORY

A baby cries for a reason. He is trying to tell you something. But when an infant is sick, the physician sometimes feels like a veterinarian: The patient can give no history, can't tell you where it hurts, actively resists examination, and bites if given the opportunity.

While the details of the infant's illness must be obtained from his mother, an older child can often give a remarkably cogent history. Sometimes I wish my middle-aged patients could stay on the track as well as some 8-year-olds.

Talk to the child! And let him talk. Give him some open-ended questions to wrestle with. "How does the pain act?" "What do you think might be causing the trouble?" You and the mother may be surprised by the history he will give.

Some injuries seem to have no cause—the black eye or twisted ankle. Maybe the child is trying to save face. Send the mother out of the room. Then try again, allowing the child a plausible excuse for not "remembering" the cause the first time. "Might you have accidentally fallen this afternoon? Were you pushed? If you were doing something wrong at the time, it doesn't interest me." "Might you have accidentally taken some of Mommy's pills?"

The child's social history is a treasury of clues, particularly if the youngster complains of headaches, stomach pains, or leg cramps. "How is school?" "Do you like school?" "Are there any problems?" "Do you get the pains during the day at school?" "Do you get them at home?"

The pediatric history often begins on the phone, requiring decisive action before the call is terminated. Hardly a month goes by that the busy family physician does not receive a call about suspected infant poisoning. When the poisoning call comes in, you and your aide should follow these rules:

1. Calm the mother and have her bring the container to the telephone.
2. Have the mother read the trade name and all ingredients, spelling those that she cannot pronounce. Write these down.
3. Instruct the mother to gag the child with her finger, trying to induce immediate vomiting—unless the child has swallowed a strong acid, alkali, or hydrocarbon.
4. Finally, instruct the mother to rush the child to your office or the hospital emergency room, bringing along the poison container.

The febrile convulsion is another telephone crisis. The mother is hysterical; it is probably the child's first convulsion, occurring during an otherwise simple febrile viral illness. The emergency treatment of the febrile convulsion—prompt reduction of the fever—should be initiated as soon as the mother hangs up the phone. Tell her to remove all the layers of blankets she has wrapped about the child (holding in the heat of the fever). Tell her to remove the clothing and wrap the convulsing youngster in damp towels. If possible, she should insert the soft tip of a man's leather belt between the child's teeth; but caution her not to get her finger between the clenched jaws, or you'll have two patients instead of one. When she has completed the emergency measures outlined above, she should rush the child to the office or emergency room.

THE PEDIATRIC EXAMINATION

In the nineteenth century, Prince Otto von Bismarck said: "You can do anything with children if you only play with them." The prince may seem an odd source of pediatric erudition, but he was right. Youngsters' visits to the doctor should have some element of fun. If gloom hangs like ether in your office, children will react accordingly. There are many ways to make the practice of pediatrics more enjoyable for patients and doctor.

The ritual recording of **height, weight, and temperature** gets the examination underway. The child who is reluctant to mount the scale to have his height measured usually offers no opposition to a wall-hung height chart (Fig. 2–1). This same scale-shy infant's weight can be determined by weighing the mother while she holds the child in her arms, then weighing the mother alone, and subtracting to find the child's weight.

Just as important as height and weight are the percentiles. Compare your patient's measurements against standard height-weight percentile charts (available from the Mead Johnson Company at no charge). The child who is in the 50th percentile for height and weight is average and trim, but young Mr. Chubby who is in the 50th percentile for height and the 95th percentile for weight has some pounds to shed.

Are your youngsters thermometer-shy? Do you worry that some spiteful 6-year-old may bite through a glass mercury-filled thermometer? Youngsters enjoy the recently developed battery-operated electronic thermometer. It requires only 15 seconds to register and, if calibrated before each reading, boasts reasonable accuracy.

Now that your office nurse has measured the height, weight, and

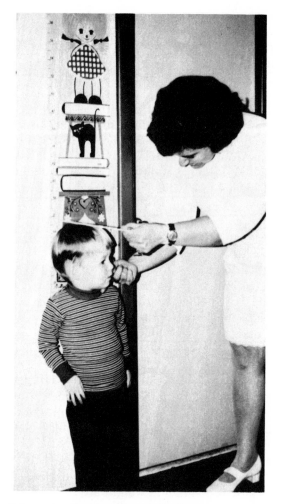

Fig. 2–1. A wall-hung height chart amuses children.

temperature, you can begin **your examination** of the youngster. No question about it—performing a satisfactory physical examination on a screaming infant is virtually impossible. Approach the pediatric patient as you would a strange animal—slowly, exuding friendship, and avoiding quick motions.

Infants, aged 18 months and younger, are probably best examined on the treatment table. In this age group, check the feet and hips first before proceeding to the abdomen. Work up the body cautiously, because the closer you get to the head and ears, the more likely the infant will begin screaming. Save the otoscopic examination for near the end, because that usually initiates crying. Once the patient begins to cry, the tonsils are usually easily visible and inguinal or umbilical hernias become obvious.

The 2- to 4-year-old child is often best examined in his mother's lap, particularly if he has an upper respiratory infection, a sore throat, or an earache. The mother's lap offers security and an extra pair of hands to restrain flailing extremities (Fig. 2–2).

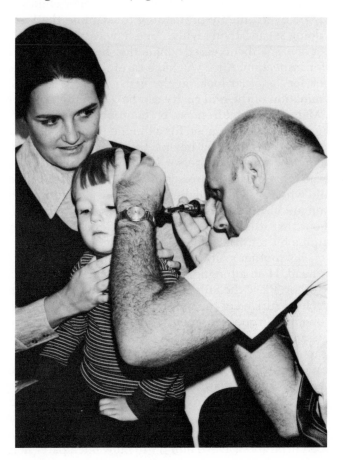

Fig. 2–2. Mother's lap offers security.

Ease into your examination, avoiding an awkward abrupt transition between history-taking and physical contact. Ask the mother to undress the child slowly while you are still talking. Hand the stethoscope head to the infant and let him hold it for a while. When you are ready to begin the examination, the youngster is already undressed and has become familiar with the stethoscope. Tell him, "That's your end of the stethoscope and this is my end. My end goes in my ears. Do you know where your end goes?" With a little coaching, most youngsters will obligingly place the stethoscope on the chest. No fuss, no crying.

The **otoscopic examination** needlessly frightens many children. Ask the older child, "Did you wash your ears today?" and he will probably offer one after the other for inspection. The younger child's otoscope-phobia may be overcome by pretending to examine the first ear (but not really doing so) and then saying, "See how easy that was. Now let's do the other one." With increased confidence, he will probably offer the other ear for inspection. After you have carefully examined the second ear, go back for "another look" at the first.

The **examination of the oral cavity** can be a gagging experience. Ask any child. Many older children can be taught to "open up the back of the throat," eliminating the need for a tongue blade. In other children, gagging can be prevented by having the child stick out his tongue, gently placing the tongue depressor in the middle of the tongue, and returning the tongue with depressor in place to the floor of the mouth. Have a child who gags at the slightest touch? Try running warm water over the tongue blade. It seems to help.

What about that stubborn 2-year-old who clenches his teeth, daring you to examine his tonsils. He has a will of iron and time is on his side. Seat him on his mother's lap and tell her to hold his hands. You can control his head. Hold a tongue depressor in one hand and your flashlight in the other. Place the fifth finger of each hand firmly on the cheek over the occlusal surface of the teeth and press in resolutely (Fig. 2–3). The child obediently opens his mouth to relieve the painful pressure of your fingers and you are afforded an excellent view of his oral cavity. It takes practice, but it works every time.

The **chest examination** may take some cunning. With the youngster still seated on his mother's lap, announce boldly, "Now we are going to listen to your heart; everyone must be very quiet." It is the rare child who will make a sound, breaking the communal vow of silence.

Do you think he is wheezing? Would you like to listen to his chest during forced expiration? Have him try to blow out a party noisemaker or the otoscope light while you listen to his lungs.

The **abdominal examination** ploy foils that screaming infant who may have abnormal abdominal findings. Every time you place him on his back, he begins to shriek. Try placing him on his hands and knees and

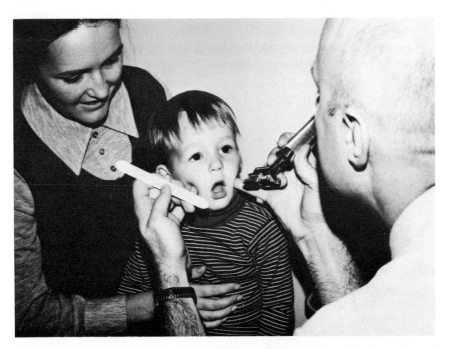

Fig. 2–3. Firm pressure with the fifth fingers opens the mouth of a reluctant child.

palpate the dependent (but now soft) abdomen with your hand under the youngster. Tenderness is just as reliable when the patient is upside down and peristalic activity sounds the same.

The adolescent with acute abdominal pain is a possible candidate for appendectomy. All such patients should be examined in the office, but sometimes the youngster is so busy guarding his painful abdomen that he can't relax for the examination. "It hurts everywhere." Talk to this youngster. Get his mind off his abdomen and onto other subjects. "How old are you?" "What grade are you in?" "Who is your teacher?" "What is your favorite subject?" "What did you do in school today?" As he begins to concentrate upon your questions, watch the abdomen relax. From then on, watch his face as you palpate. It will tell more than his verbal responses.

Of course, the prudent physician will not initiate his abdominal examination by mashing hard on the right lower quadrant. Lay your hand gently on the abdomen. Let the temperature difference between hand and abdomen equalize, and let the patient get used to the feel of your examining fingers on his abdominal wall. Then begin to palpate gently, beginning with an apparently pain-free area. Save the deep palpation of the tender spot until last.

Think he's reacting to your hand and not the pain? Try listening to the abdomen with your stethoscope and unobtrusively depress the 'scope head, in fact, deeply palpating the abdomen in that area (Fig. 2–4). The child with true tenderness will quickly report his displeasure with your maneuver.

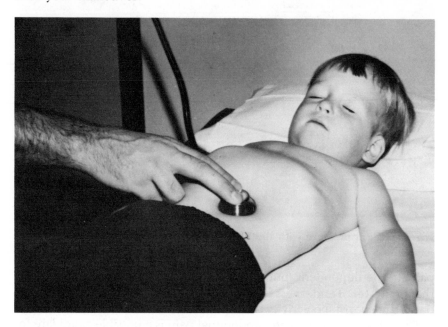

Fig. 2–4. Abdominal palpation with the stethoscope head.

The **rectal examination** is often indicated in infants and children. A rectal examination is (or should be) performed immediately on all newborn infants by the obstetrician. When performing the rectal examination in your office, reassure the child and mother that your examining finger is no larger than the youngster's normal bowel movements, then proceed gently.

The **totally unmanageable youngster** is mercifully uncommon. He bites, kicks, and spits. No one is going to examine him! Usually this child is reacting for the benefit of his mother. Send her out of the room, but don't call for help. You shouldn't need it. Tell the young hellion what you intend to do, that it *will be done*, and that the examination will be completed. Firmly assume control of the relationship. Then proceed as though there were no question about his cooperation. This child really does not care about your opinion of him and will usually not react for your benefit.

If this fails, with the mother still out of the room, restrain him and do what needs to be done.

PEDIATRIC DIAGNOSIS AND TREATMENT

"A smart mother makes often a better diagnosis than a poor doctor" said August Bier (1861–1949). Right he was! And the more offspring a mother has, the better diagnostician she becomes. Pay attention to your smart mothers; you can learn a lot of pediatrics from them.

Teething can cause fever, contrary to popular medical misconception. Ask any mother. But you should ascribe fever to teething only after a thorough physical examination has ruled out other causes. Can anything be done for teething? Don't forget the therapeutic value of baby aspirin, a cold teething ring, and an anesthetic solution such as Xylocaine Viscous.

As you ponder your dazzling diagnostic acumen and therapeutic triumphs, remind your ego that up to 75 percent of sick children in your office suffer from nonspecific, **self-limited viral infections.** Be as clever as you care to, differentiating ECHOvirus infections from fifth disease, but don't succumb to the temptation to overtreat your patients. In self-limited infections, any medication works. Use the inexpensive, nonallergenic, safe ones.

While on the topic of medicine, are you familiar with the Flexidose spoon, a test-tube-shaped plastic spoon with a long sipping lip?

A child with **severe gastroenteritis** often vomits all medicine and fluids. The medication can be administered rectally or by injection. But what about fluids? Try popsicles. Tasty, cold, and dissolved slowly in the mouth, the fluids from the popsicle rarely upset the stomach. The youngster who regurgitates all fluids will sometimes retain Coca-Cola syrup in water.

The **umbilical hernia,** seen through mother's eyes, is a grotesque disfiguring appendage. "Doctor, the baby's grandmother says I should tape a silver dollar over that umbilical hernia." Don't do it. Explain that taping an umbilical hernia will only lead to adhesive dermatitis of the abdominal wall. Virtually every umbilical hernia will close by the time the infant is 2 or 3 years old. Reassure the mother by letting her feel the hernia ring; then ceremoniously measure its diameter at each visit, documenting the gradual closure.

Milk babies abound. "My baby is a good eater, doctor. He takes 2 qt of milk a day. He just doesn't like solid food." Preposterous? Not a bit. Doctors hear this story frequently from otherwise intelligent mothers. Of course, the infant is a classic milk baby—fat and pudgy, but pale because of iron-deficiency anemia. Milk is a poor source of iron. Treat this child by rigidly restricting the milk intake to 28 oz daily. Correct the anemia with supplemental oral iron. Once his milk consumption is limited, the child's appetite for solid food will improve miraculously.

Reading difficulties, educators tell us, can be caused by mixed dominance—a lack of clear-cut right- or left-handedness. You may be called upon to determine laterality in your elementary grade youngsters. Check right- or left-handedness by tossing the child a wad of paper; see which hand he uses to throw it back. Check visual dominance by handing him a sheet of paper with a hole in the center. Tell him, "Look at me through the hole." See which eye he uses.

THE OVERWEIGHT CHILD

Adolescent obesity is caused by systematic overfeeding of the child. The problem probably began in infancy, the mother equating food and love. Now the unhappy obese adolescent looks to the icebox for security.

How to reduce this chubby cherub? Don't waste your time and the mother's money if the child is not interested. The primary motivation must come from the youngster. When the child fervently wishes to be slim and is willing to "do anything," the battle is half won.

During the weight-reduction program of an overweight adolescent, the whole family must diet. It is not fair to give the others fattening casseroles and desserts while the overweight youngster is restricted to lettuce and cottage cheese. As a matter of practical fact, the parents of overweight adolescents can usually benefit from a low-calorie diet.

I have found a weight reduction program that works quite well if the patient will cooperate. No pills. No shots. Just a detailed diet diary. The patient is given a simplified 1000-calorie diet outline and a list of the caloric content of all common foods. Then he or she can plan a diet, recording everything eaten at each meal or between meals, and totaling the caloric values at the day's end.

The child returns to the office for ritual weighing every 2 or 3 weeks and presents the diet diary for inspection. Indiscretions are criticized and weight loss is praised. Some of the diets recorded by 10- and 12-year-old girls have been classic nutritional programs, as good as any professional could plan. But for the plan to succeed, the child must keep the diary, not the mother.

Try this method on your hefty preteens. In fact, it works well at all ages. I have one 55-year-old gentleman who makes a 150-calorie allowance for his predinner drink each evening.

THE PARTING SHOT

Shots hurt! The fear of an injection colors a child's responses whenever he is in the doctor's office. Keep this in mind and you will understand why children act as they often do.

Don't let the mother tell the child the shot isn't going to hurt. And don't you do it. (I sometimes jokingly tell the child the shot isn't going to hurt *me* a bit.) The penalty for deception is a twisting, startled, disappointed youngster who has suddenly found Mommy doesn't always tell the truth.

Anticipation of the injection is as painful as the shot itself, and once an injection is mentioned, finish the job promptly before the child panics.

Prepare the injection out of the child's sight. Don't allow him to watch you fill a syringe that he knows full well will shortly be plunged into his tender bottom.

Have a really needle-shy patient? Spank the area sharply before injecting the needle. Or spray a whiff of ethyl chloride to "freeze the skin."

As he leaves, be sure to tell the youngster that he was a good patient. Who knows? Next time he may be.

References and Suggestions for Further Reading

1. Alpert J J: Effective use of comprehensive pediatric care. Am J Dis Child 116:-529–533, 1968.
2. Alpert J J, Kosa J, Haggerty R J: Attitudes and satisfactions of low-income families receiving comprehensive pediatric care. J Public Health 60:499–506, 1970.
3. Chess S: Individuality in children, its importance to the pediatrician. J Pediatr 69:-676–684, 1966.
4. Cooke R E: The Biologic Basis of Pediatric Practice. New York, McGraw-Hill, 1968.
5. Faigel H C: Small expectations: The vulnerable child syndrome. GP 34:78–84, 1966.

6.   Gibson E J: Principles of Perceptual Learning and Development. New York, Appleton, 1969.

7.   Krugman S, Ward R: Infectious Diseases of Children, 4th ed. St Louis, Mosby, 1968.

8.   Nelson W E, Vaughan C, McKay J R: Textbook of Pediatrics. Philadelphia, Saunders, 1969.

9.   Phansalkar S V, Holt L E Jr: Observations on the immediate treatment of poisoning. J Pediatr 72:683–684, 1968.

10.   Rees G J: Intensive therapy in pediatrics. Br Med J 2:1611–1616, 1966.

11.   Report to the President: White House Conference on Children. Washington, D C, GPO, 1970.

12.   Schiff G M, Bloom J E: Evaluation of rubella vaccination in large school system. J Pediatr 78:211–219, 1971.

13.   Steele R W, Tanaka P T, Lara R P, Bass J W: Evaluation of sponging and of oral antipyretic therapy to reduce fever. J Pediatr 77:824–829, 1970.

14.   Wagner R F: Dyslexia and Your Child: A Guide for Teachers and Parents. New York, Harper & Row, 1971.

15.   White K L: Future forms of medical care for children. Am J Dis Child 116:458–498, 1968.

16.   Wingert W A, Friedman D B, Larson W R: Pediatric emergency room patient. Am J Dis Child 115:48–56, 1968.

3

Everyday Ear, Nose, and Throat Problems

Nature has given man one tongue, but two ears, that we may hear twice as much as we speak.

Epictetus
(60–120)

The ear, nose, and throat, with their maze of hidden cavities, are the sites of many problems of everyday medical practice. Curiously, we spend years treating elusive afflictions of the paranasal sinuses, the mastoid sinuses, the eustachian tubes, the middle ear cavity, the inner ear, and the nasopharynx, but rarely examine these structures in the living patient. The doctor relies heavily upon the patient's symptoms, examines those areas that are accessible, makes his diagnosis often by inference, and prescribes as best he can with the therapeutic alternatives at his disposal.

EVERYDAY EAR PROBLEMS

The function of the ear is hearing. Keep this in mind when you treat diseases of the ear. The ear canal may be as smooth as a baby's bottom, and the eardrum may glisten like morning dew on grass, but if the patient can't hear, your brilliant diagnosis and therapy have been of little help to him. In my practice, all patients with ear disorders are followed by screening audiometry, and this procedure is also part of my routine physical examination for adults and children. It yields valuable baseline data that become important when ear disease strikes. The screening audiometer is battery-operated and costs about $100. Audiometry is as important in the evaluation of ear disorders as is the testing of visual acuity in diseases of the eye. The nurse performs the test, which takes about 2 minutes of her time.

The child with **acute otitis media** characteristically shows a hearing loss, most marked in the high frequencies. Following therapy with an antibiotic, a decongestant, and possibly nosedrops, the youngster is reexamined at weekly intervals until the eardrum returns to normal and the hearing reaches its pretreatment level.

When rechecking a child who is being treated for otitis media, word your questions carefully. If you ask him if he has pain, the child experiencing a sensation of pressure will reply, "No." I often ask the child, "Which ear had the earache last week?" The child who can't remember which ear was sore is probably having no distress now.

Ask the mother how the child adjusts the audio volume of the television; it's more reliable than her assessment of how well the child hears what she says. Some children with normal hearing suffer from acute inattention. A child with a high-frequency hearing loss hears the father's deeper voice well but has difficulty with the mother's higher pitched speech.

Some days seem to be spent **removing things from ears.** The most common offender is earwax. Excessive cerumen commonly blocks hearing in adults, and its removal is indicated. The condition is less common in children, and the fortuitous finding of wax in the ear by the school nurse does not justify its removal. Wax in the ear is normal and rarely becomes inspissated in children.

Before you syringe the ear, instill a few drops of Debrox (with the patient lying on his side so the drops don't run out), and go see another patient for a few minutes. While you are gone, the Debrox will loosen the cerumen. Then draw a basin of water about body temperature (cold water in the ear causes vertigo). Since a little water always gets away from you during ear syringing, gown the patient with a waterproof drape. I use a fetching black cape donated by a local beautician, but a local dental supplier may have a more clinical model.

Syringe the ear gently. In most cases, your efforts will be rewarded by the dislodgment of a firm plug of cerumen and the sudden return of the patient's hearing. Don't lose your patience if the plug is stubborn. Give the patient a prescription for Debrox and instruct him to instill a few drops in the ear every 2 hours while he is awake; try syringing again 2 days later.

If only wax were the only thing that clogged ear canals. I have removed cellophane, peanuts, Play-Doh, and even an imitation pearl from ears.

Someday you will encounter the patient with a live insect in his ear. Resist the temptation to flood the ear with water, bloating the insect's body into an irretrievable mass of soggy protoplasm. If you take the telephone call, tell the patient to try the following maneuver at home: Pull the external ear up and back to open the ear canal; then shine a flashlight into the opening. The insect, attracted to the light, will often gratefully escape. Success is not invariable, however. Ten minutes later the patient is in your office. The insect showed no interest in the light and continues to flutter against the eardrum. Fill the ear canal with mineral oil or Auralgan to drown the insect. Then under direct observation remove the remains with a ring curette or forceps.

Then there is the foreign body in the ear that resists syringing and has no handles to grasp with forceps. It can usually be removed with a suction catheter. Cut the end of a straight urethral catheter flat. Insert it in the ear canal and use suction by mouth to withdraw the foreign body (Fig. 3–1).

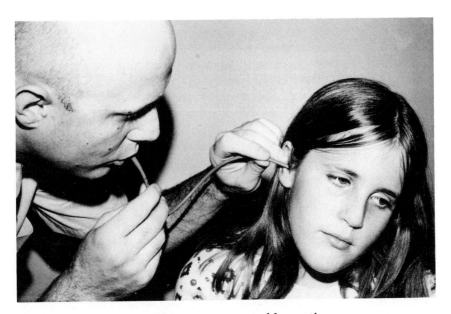

Fig. 3–1. A foreign body in the ear is removed by suction.

Another vexing ear problem is **recurrent labyrinthine vertigo,** often resistant to your most diligent medical therapy. Tell your patient to try this technique: Find the motion that most frequently results in vertigo and purposely induce attacks as often as possible. This reduces the brain's vulnerability to abnormal impulses from the receptor organs, much as graduated allergy injections reduce susceptibility to the allergen.

EVERYDAY NOSE PROBLEMS

If there is any doubt as to whether a person is or is not dead, apply lightly roasted onion to his nostrils, and if he is alive, he will immediately scratch his nose.

John of Mirfield
(1362–1407)

Like his ears, the child's nose is the repository for a wide variety of **foreign objects**—corn, peas, wheat, barley, and toys. Be suspicious of the child with a unilateral purulent nasal discharge; it is probably caused by a foreign body.

Mercifully, most nasal foreign bodies can be removed by forceps if the child is restrained, the naris properly illuminated, and the object exposed with a nasal speculum. Be careful. You may not get a second chance. Fragment the foreign body or push it further back and you're in trouble. Sometimes a good sneeze solves the problem. Try blowing cigar smoke in the child's nose, while covering his mouth to force the ensuing sneeze out the nose.

Nosebleeds, like babies, often come in the middle of the night. Oh, for a way to treat nosebleeds without struggling with a blood-soaked nasal pack at 3 A.M.! Of course, you told the patient to lie down and apply pressure with a clean handkerchief for 15 minutes, but this didn't work. (You suspect the patient kept peeking to see if the bleeding had stopped.) Tell him to clamp a common clothespin on his nose and leave it in place for several hours, unless severely painful. The properly placed clothespin applies pressure directly at Little's area and will arrest many a nosebleed.

I have long used carbazochrome salicylate (Adrenosem) in the office and home treatment of nosebleed. Adrenosem reduces capillary bleeding, and 10 mg is administered intramuscularly to the acute nosebleed victim. Patients with recurrent nosebleeds are advised to keep Adrenosem tablets at home. At the first sign of nosebleed, two 2.5-mg tablets should be taken, then one tablet every 4 hours until the nose-bleed ceases.

In some cases, all these efforts fail, and then the physician has no alternative but to get out of bed whatever the hour, drive to the patient's house, and pack his nose.

How about the patient who **can't smell** or who suffers **distortion of odors.** These conditions are often caused by chronic allergic congestion of the nasal membranes. Consultation with an allergist, followed by skin testing and appropriate desensitization, may bring relief to the patient.

The patient who thinks he has a **broken nose** probably has. Don't guess about nasal fractures. Free breathing through both nostrils is laudable but is an unreliable diagnostic sign in suspected nasal fractures. External swelling can obscure the injury, and a few weeks later when the swelling subsides the deformity you missed will be obvious. Get an x-ray! And avoid the embarrassment of overlooking a nasal fracture buried under soft tissue swelling.

EVERYDAY MOUTH AND THROAT PROBLEMS

Tongue-tie is not uncommon in infants and children. Often encountered in the newborn baby, the tight lingular frenulum should be snipped unceremoniously. The necessary equipment for the procedure includes a tongue-tie director, sharp scissors, and a nurse to steady the infant's head.

Occasionally a tight tongue-tie escapes notice until the child enters school; then it is manifest as impaired speech with specific difficulty in pronouncing consonants. The tongue-tie is easily corrected in the office. Inject 1 ml of 2% lidocaine (Xylocaine) into the frenulum, elevate the tongue with the tongue-tie director, and carefully snip the membrane. Avoid cutting the artery at the base of the membrane; if you cut it, a suture will be required to control bleeding.

A common Saturday night dental emergency is the **bleeding tooth socket** that follows an extraction within the past 48 hours. Instruct the patient to moisten an ordinary tea bag and place it in the socket, exerting some pressure with the opposing teeth. The tannic acid of the tea hastens blood clotting, and the mechanical pressure on the tea bag staunches the flow of blood.

Should Johnny have his tonsils out? Questions concerning tonsillectomy arise almost daily during the winter months. Increasing evidence indicates that the tonsils play an important but not vital role in immunity and development of facial structures. But, as with any expendable organ, when disease renders the part a liability to the body, it should be sacrificed mercilessly. The child who has five or six episodes of tonsillitis or otitis media during a calendar year is a good candidate for tonsillectomy. Enlarged adenoids cause mouth breathing and snoring, relative indications for adenoidectomy. Elephantine tonsils, pocked with crypts, may meet in the midline and hinder swallowing of meat and vegetables. Following tonsillectomy, look for this child to gain weight rapidly.

The frequent occurrence of common colds is in no way an indication for tonsillectomy, and if the operation is performed for no more valid reason, the physician will continue to treat a tonsilless child for frequent common colds.

Aphthous ulcers cause pain disproportionate to the apparent lesion and frequently bring the patient to the office. Try light cautery with a silver nitrate stick followed by the local application of Gly-Oxide four times daily. If nutrition is a problem in a child with aphthous stomatitis, prescribe popsicles or frozen Kool-Aid on a stick: The cold anesthetizes the oral mucosa and the fluid maintains hydration.

Dislocation of the temporomandibular joint can be hazardous to the neophyte physician attempting reduction with his unprotected thumbs. Before depressing the mandibular molars, wrap your thumbs generously with gauze or, better yet, don your leaded x-ray gloves (Fig. 3–2).

Laceration of the throat, usually caused by a lollipop stick, rarely requires surgical repair. Most are simple puncture wounds and need only sustained pressure for a few minutes to arrest bleeding. Reassurance and a tetanus toxoid booster complete the therapy. Discourage repeated inspection of the area; the action of saliva turns the ragged wound margins a dirty gray, making the injury appear more serious than it is.

The suspected fish bone in the throat can be an elusive problem. Laryngoscopy is unremarkable, but the patient insists the bone is still there. Have him swallow a cotton ball saturated with barium. The barium-soaked cotton ball will (or should) snag on the offending fish bone, marking the site like a beacon on x-ray examination.

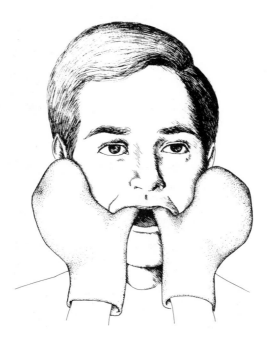

Fig. 3–2. **Leaded x-ray gloves protect thumbs during reduction of a dislocated temporomandibular joint.**

ALLERGIC DISORDERS OF THE EAR, NOSE, AND THROAT

The allergic salute, an extended forefinger passing under the nose, is the unmistakable sign of an allergy sufferer, like a recognition signal between conspirators (Fig. 3–3).

Household pets protect the home, help youngsters learn responsibility, and cause thousands of cases of respiratory allergy. The sniffing, sneezing, wheezing patient will dustproof the home, install air conditioning, or move to Arizona before he will part with his four-legged friend. How many allergic children do you know who have a dog and two cats sleeping on the bed? If the allergic symptoms are severe enough for the patient to consider skin testing and desensitization, they are serious enough to warrant a trial of life without Rover. Persuade your patient to board his pet for 2 weeks in a kennel, vacuum the house to remove all dog (or cat) dander, and see how much better he feels. "Now shouldn't you find another home for your pet?"

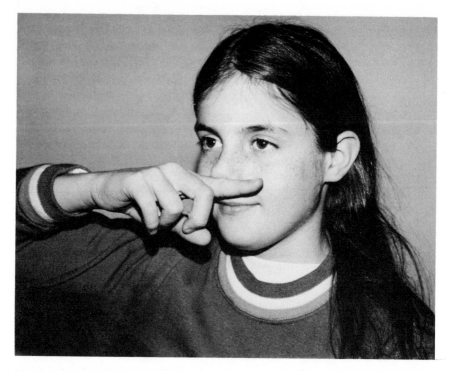

Fig. 3–3. The allergic salute.

Mold allergies are common, often tucked in incidentally with the diagnosis of multiple other allergies. Mold? Who has mold? The allergy sufferer may. Check the water basin in that new humidifier, and you may be surprised to find a thriving community of mold.

House dust allergies are easy to diagnose. All houses have dust. New houses have sawdust and plaster dust. Old houses have dust accumulated over the years (undoubtedly due to previous owners). Forced-air furnaces relentlessly circulate dust from one part of the house to another, but these same air ducts lend themselves to easy filtration of the air. Don't use muslin: It's too thick. Stretch material from an old pair of pantyhose under the grate in each room. The porous material effectively filters small particles but allows a free flow of air.

Skin testing of the allergic patient pinpoints the allergen. Repeat skin testing following desensitization documents the response to therapy. But memory is short, and words don't do justice to the wheal and flare. How to compare reactions from one year to the next? Write the name of the test material on the skin next to each reaction. Outline the wheal with your skin-marking pencil. Then photograph the area for your records. Not a camera buff? Then outline the wheal with a ballpoint pen and cover the area with Scotch Magic Transparent Tape. When you lift the tape, you will find that enough ink is lifted to accurately transfer the outline to your records. Don't try this on hairy areas or you will have shaggy records. With visual evidence before you, year-by-year comparison is easy.

References and Suggestions for Further Reading

1. Ballenger H C: Diseases of the Nose, Throat, and Ear, 11th ed. Philadelphia, Lea & Febiger, 1969.
2. Banaszak E F, Thiede W H, Fink J N: Hypersensitivity pneumonitis due to contamination of air conditioner. N Engl J Med 283:271–276, 1970.
3. Bierman C W, Pierson W E, Donaldson J A: The evaluation of middle ear function in children. Am J Dis Child 120:233–236, 1970.
4. Brown E B, Clavery O, Carol B: Diagnosis of allergy. NY State J Med 71:845–847, 1971.
5. Brownlee R C Jr, DeLoache W R, Cowan C C Jr: Otitis media in children: Incidence, treatment and prognosis in pediatric practice. J Pediatr 75:636–642, 1969.
6. Catlin F I, de Haan V: Tongue tie. Arch Otolaryngol 94:548–557, 1971.
7. Committee on Conservation of Hearing of the American Academy of Ophthalmology and Otolaryngology. Standard classification for surgery of chronic ear infection. Trans Am Acad Ophthalmol Otolaryngol 69: 332–334, 1965.
8. Cortese T A Jr, Dickey R A: Complications of ear piercing. Am Fam Physician GP 4:66–72, 1971.
9. Hagy G W: Prognosis of positive allergy skin tests in asymptomatic population. J Allergy 48:200–211, 1971.
10. Lenihan J M A, Christie J F, Russell T S, Orr N M, Hamilton D, Knox E C: The threshold of hearing in school children. J Laryngol Otol 58:375–385, 1971.
11. Mitchell D F, Standish S M, Fast T B: Oral Diagnosis/Oral Medicine. Philadelphia, Lea & Febiger, 1971.
12. Norman P S, Winkenwerder W L, Lichtenstein L M: Maintenance immunotherapy in ragweed hay fever. J Allergy 47:273–282, 1971.
13. Rapaport H G, Linde S M: The Complete Allergy Guide. New York, Simon & Schuster, 1971.
14. Scott-Brown W G: Diseases of the Ear, Nose, and Throat. London, Butterworth, 1965.

4

In the Twinkling of an Eye

Our sight is the most perfect and the most delightful of all our senses.

Joseph Addison
June 21, 1712

No craftsman will ever devise a camera to equal the human eye, the aperture adjusting and focus changing constantly, recording retinal images during all the waking hours. But illnesses and injuries of the eye abound. Accurate diagnosis, prompt therapy, and careful follow-up are imperative.

EXAMINATION OF THE EYE

The **visual acuity** should be recorded in all cases of eye complaints and, indeed, on routine physical examinations. A well-illuminated Snellen eye chart is indispensable to the doctor's office. Most offices have a hallway at least 20 ft long with a wall or door at one end that can hold the chart. A 20-ft distance marker should be placed on the floor. I use a bronze door plate, with the words "20 feet" inscribed in the space conventionally allotted to "Smith" or "Jones." If you don't have a 20-ft hall, use a 10-ft Snellen chart, available in a package that includes self-contained fluorescent lights behind translucent panels.

Visual acuity in children aged 4 and over can be accurately determined with the proper eye chart and patience. An E chart can be used. Tell the child the E is a dog sitting on its hind legs and ask, "Which way is the dog pointing?"

Some children respond to picture charts with progressively smaller line drawings of stars, boats, and circles. Most youngsters can accurately name these common symbols, but let the child view the chart at close range before testing, so that you agree on the names to be used.

The child's attention fatigues quickly. Don't try to have him identify every symbol in every line. Skip down the chart until you find the smallest line he can name confidently. Make it a game and offer a prize (a ring or plastic car) if he cooperates.

The **conjunctiva and cornea** are examined with a loupe and a light. Use oblique illumination to detect corneal irregularities. Side illumination allows estimation of the depth of an anterior chamber. Depress the lower eyelid to view the palpebral conjunctiva, after you have made sure the patient is not wearing contact lenses. Don't make the mistake of beginning your examination by depressing the lower lid and flipping the contact lens onto the floor.

Evert the upper eyelid by depressing the base of the tarsal plate with an applicator stick, flipping the lid up on itself. Only a freshman medical student would pretend to examine the upper palpebral conjunctiva without lid eversion. Here is where most foreign bodies hide; they can be easily removed with a moist cotton-tipped applicator.

The **chambers and ocular fundus** are examined with the ophthalmo-scope—an important instrument in the diagnosis of many ocular and systemic conditions. Begin by focusing on the cornea, looking for irregularity or abrasion; then progressively focus through the chambers, noting any cloudiness; then focus on the retina, describing the important structures there. Most adults can hold their eyes steady during funduscopic examination, but how about children? Give the child an object on the far wall to focus on—a calendar or coat hook. Then tell him, "My head is going to get in the way, but keep looking through my head and pretend you still see the calendar. Try not to look at the light." Then look fast, before the child loses interest in the game.

Tonometry should be performed as part of the routine physical examination of all persons over the age of 40. A reliable tonometer costs about $30; its use is speedy, painless, and easy to learn. If you haven't learned how to use a tonometer during medical school and internship, your local ophthalmologist will be flattered to instruct you. During tonometry, the patient must hold his eyes steady. Stick a colored thumbtack in the ceiling over the head of your examination table and tell the patient to focus on it with the eye that is not being examined.

Both eyes should be kept open. Restrain the eyelids with gentle pressure on the bony margins, but avoid pressure on the globe that would elevate the reading (Fig. 4–1). I prefer proparacaine hydrochloride (Ophthaine) as a topical anesthetic. Reassure the patient that his vision will not be blurred following its use.

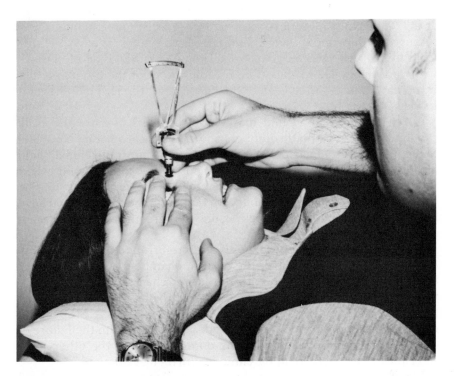

Fig. 4–1. Ocular tonometry.

DIAGNOSIS OF EYE DISEASE

The **red eye** is the classic problem in differential diagnosis of eye disease: Possibilities include conjunctivitis, uveitis-iritis, or glaucoma. Note the patient's age: Glaucoma is uncommon under age 40. Check his visual acuity: Conjunctivitis should not impair vision. Note the character of the pain: Is it the scratchy discomfort of conjunctivitis or the severe unremitting deep pain of more severe ocular pathology? Is the palpebral conjunctiva injected, a reassuring sign of conjunctivitis? Are the chambers clear when viewed with the ophthalmoscope or is the cloudiness of uveitis present? Does an elevated ocular tension indicate glaucoma? All pink eyes are not pinkeye.

The **lazy eye** is a popular descriptive term for imbalance of the extraocular muscles of the eye resulting in a failure of convergence. Binocular vision produces a double image, and the child's mind "shuts off" one eye. Failure to diagnose the lazy eye in a preschool child results in loss of central vision in the shut-off eye. A specialist's problem? Not at all! That child may never get to the ophthalmologist unless you suspect the disorder and refer him. The lazy eye test is easy. Tell the child to keep his eyes on your nose. Then block the vision of one eye with your hand. There should be no adjustment of the other eye, but if you have blocked the vision of the "good" eye, the lazy eye will shift to focus at that time.

Color blindness in a child may elude diagnosis because the child cannot read the schematic numbers on pseudoisochromatic plates. Obtain a few lengths of yarn of various colors, cut the strands in half, and arrange them in two identical piles. Be sure you have included bright red and green hues. Ask the child to match the colors in each pile. The color-blind child will have trouble with reds and greens. Think you have found a color-blind girl? Check again. Red-green color blindness is exceedingly rare in females.

The child with **reading problems** is often referred to the physician by the school. You should check the cornea, chambers, and retina carefully; determine near vision with the Jaeger chart; and then measure visual acuity. Here you may find a clue. The youngster may read the 20/20 line confidently but, unprompted, from right to left. Suspect the child of mixed dominance—a reading disability related to the failure of one cerebral hemisphere to assume dominance over the other—and refer him to a special reading clinic for further evaluation.

Floaters are concretions in the vitreous, common in myopia, and usually harmless. But watch out! A sudden shower of floaters may signal the onset of retinal detachment. Suspect this particularly in diabetic or hypertensive patients. Ask if there has been partial loss of vision in the involved eye, perhaps "like pulling down a window shade." Examine the retina carefully, but don't be surprised if the funduscopic examination is unremarkable in early disease. Check the visual fields, using the classic maneuver of a wiggling finger or bright object entering the peripheral field of vision. Check all quadrants of each eye. Any visual field loss in one or more quadrants should raise suspicion. Refer this patient to an ophthalmologist immediately. You make the call, or the answering service may schedule him for the middle of next month.

MANAGEMENT OF EYE INJURIES

Foreign Bodies are attracted to the eye like crows to a corn field. Most foreign bodies are trapped under the tarsal plate of the upper lid or embedded in the cornea. Following careful examination of the globe, instill a few drops of Ophthaine and evert the upper lid, wiping away any offending foreign body. The particle embedded in the cornea is more difficult. Wiping with a cotton-tipped applicator may push it in further. Try flushing the eye with sterile distilled water. Metal objects can sometimes be removed with a special eye magnet. Most corneal foreign bodies, however, require removal with an eye spud or a 20-gauge needle. Adequate magnification and illumination are essential. Watch out for the rust ring that quickly forms around steel particles; this should be removed by an ophthalmologist following slit-lamp examination. Once the foreign particle has been removed, patch the eye securely and instruct the patient to return for reexamination tomorrow, but admonish him to call promptly if severe symptoms develop in the meantime.

The **corneal abrasion** verifies the English proverb "A small hurt in the eye is a great one." Tiny babies have disabled their fathers by brushing a fingernail across Daddy's cornea. During hunting season, you will probably be visited by a few intrepid hunters who have walked into tree branches. Small boys throwing stones account for a high percentage of corneal abrasions. Most corneal abrasions can be identified with adequate magnification and oblique illumination; elusive ones can be visualized by staining with fluorescein. A few drops of Ophthaine will facilitate examination and allow detection of impaired visual acuity.

Most clean corneal abrasions heal uneventfully in a few days with no more treatment than simple patching to keep the eye closed day and night. If infection is suspected, have the patient instill 2 drops of chloramphenicol (Chloromycetin) 0.5% eyedrops hourly while awake. Corneal abrasions are painful, so don't forget to prescribe an analgesic, such as propoxyphene (Darvon), one 65-mg capsule every 4 hours as needed. Be wary of the corneal abrasion directly over the pupil; there is no margin for error here. And be suspicious of the tree-branch-scratched cornea; it is usually dirtier than you estimate. I refer a high percentage of branch-scratched corneas to the ophthalmologist.

Check the corneal abrasion daily until it heals, even if this means a Sunday visit. Warn the patient to call promptly if his symptoms become worse. Don't succumb to the patient's pleadings for a prescription for those wonderful anesthetic eyedrops you used in the office; serious damage can occur to the anesthetized eye.

Penetrating foreign bodies of the eye are foolers. A chip from the head of a hammer may have made a tiny hole as it penetrated the globe, even though it has produced minimal local redness and pain. The steel fragment is there and can result in permanent total loss of vision in an eye which appears barely injured when first examined. Be suspicious of the high-impact eye injury. If you expected to find a foreign body and didn't, why not? Where could it be? Don't forget the value of x-rays in detecting the presence of radiopaque foreign bodies. Are you in doubt? X-rays inconclusive or unavailable? Then gently patch the eye and refer the patient to an ophthalmologist.

TREATMENT OF EYE DISEASE

Patching palliates the diseased eye. The emergency treatment of most eye injuries includes careful patching. The patient with Bell's palsy, who cannot voluntarily close his eye, needs patching to preserve the integrity of the corneal epithelium. Sometimes a simple eye patch will not keep the eye closed. In these cases, a small wad of gauze or cotton under the patch will exert just enough pressure to keep the upper lid closed. Or, particularly in patients with Bell's palsy, try a single Steri-Strip placed vertically to hold the lids together (Fig. 4–2).

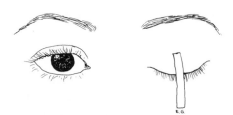

Fig. 4–2. A vertically placed Steri-Strip holds eyelids together and prevents corneal damage in Bell's palsy or stroke.

In elderly patients **corneal irritation** can result from inversion of the lower lid which allows eyelashes to rub against the cornea. These patients can use Steri-Strips or Scotch Magic Transparent Tape to hold the lower lid in proper position.

Contact lenses can contribute to chronic conjunctivitis. That vain young woman who visits your office repeatedly with conjunctival infections must forsake her contact lenses for at least several weeks to allow the epithelium to heal without the recurrent irritation of these foreign bodies.

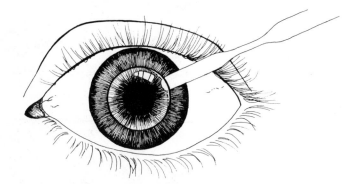

Fig. 4–3. A stuck contact lens is removed with an eye spud.

Do you know how to remove a contact lens that is stuck because a suction seal has formed between the lens and the cornea? Anesthetize the eye with Ophthaine; then pry up the lens with an eye spud or a 20-gauge needle (Fig. 4–3). Sometimes a sudden burst of air from an empty syringe will dislodge the stuck contact lens. Once the lens is removed, advise the patient not to replace it for at least 24 hours.

Eyedrops terrify children. That huge drop seems to bombard the eye like a cannonball, and the child can only lie there and watch helplessly. Here's the secret of the peaceful instillation of eyedrops in children: Ask the child to lie flat on his back and to close both eyes tightly; then instill 3 drops of the ophthalmic solution at the inner canthus of the eye (Fig. 4–4). With the child still lying face up, tell him he may now open his eyes. As the eyes open, the drops run in painlessly.

Eye ointments have the advantage of longer contact with the epithelium. The proper application of eye ointments involves pulling down the lower lid, instilling a thin ribbon of ointment inside the lower lid, and then allowing the lid to fall back in place, distributing the ointment throughout the eye. Eye ointments cause blurring of the vision, and during your years of practice, you will find patients prefer ophthalmic solutions.

Ophthalmic solutions and ointments are both rapidly removed from the eyes. Tears bathe the eyes constantly, rapidly washing your medication down the nasolacrimal duct. For your ophthalmic prescription to

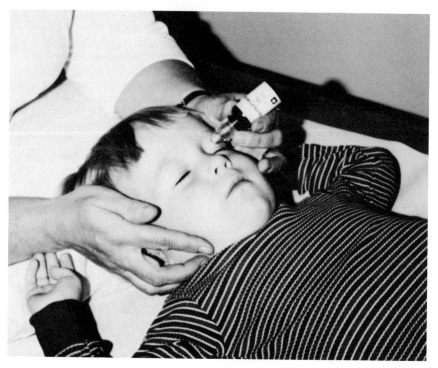

Fig. 4–4. Atraumatic method of administering eyedrops to a child.

be of value, it must be applied frequently—every hour or two while the patient is awake.

References and Suggestions for Further Reading

1. Blodi F: What's new in ophthalmology. Med Times 99:73–79, 1971.

2. Brindley G S: Physiology of the Retina and Visual Pathway. Baltimore, Williams & Wilkins, 1970.

3. Buxton J N, Locke C R: Therapeutic evaluation of hydrophilic contact lenses. Am J Ophthalmol 72:532–535, 1971.

4. Hauser W A: Incidence and prognosis of Bell's palsy in the population of Rochester, Minnesota. Mayo Clin Proc 46:258–264, 1971.

5. Kaufman R S: Health hazards in industrial welding. JAMA 216:677–678, 1971.

6. Kolker A E, Hetherington J Jr: Becker-Schaffer's Diagnosis and Therapy of the Glaucomas. St Louis, Mosby, 1970.

7. Law and medicine: Foreign bodies in the eye. JAMA 218:495–496, 1971.

8. Mustarde J C, Jones L T, Callahan A: Ophthalmic Plastic Surgery Up to Date. Birmingham, Ala, Aesculapius, 1970.

9. Neumann E: A review of four hundred cases of vernal conjunctivitis. Am J Ophthalmol 47:166–171, 1959.

10. Sheldon G M: Misuse of corneal anesthetics. Can Med Assoc J 104:528–534, 1971.

11. Thygeson P, Kimura S J: Chronic conjunctivitis. Trans Am Acad Ophthalmol Otolaryngol 67:494–517, 1963.

12. Trotter R R: Cornea and sclera. Arch Ophthalmol 79:338–342, 1968.

5

Internal Medicine: The Science of Detection

Medicine is a science of uncertainty and an art of probability.

Sir William Osler
(1849–1919)

Internal medicine lacks the drama of surgery and the clamor of pediatrics. But softly, with seductive hints and quiet glances, she entices the doctor into the intrigue of diagnosis. And in the end, when least expected, she tells her secrets in a whisper.

RESPIRATORY DISEASE

Chronic pulmonary disease is a leading cause of respiratory distress. As Chevalier Jackson said, "All that wheezes is not asthma." Chronic bronchitis is another cause of wheezing.

Where does chronic bronchitis come from? Your patient will fervently condemn auto exhaust fumes and vividly describe the musty odor at work, but what about the one or two packs of cigarettes he smokes daily? That's his problem! Can you get him to stop smoking for his lungs' sake? Fear seems to motivate a patient to cease smoking only when linked to a specific occurrence, such as a heart attack or pneumonia. Reducing his daily consumption of cigarettes may work for a while, but the next time the patient faces a crisis, he will be smoking two packs a day again.

When Cortez landed in Mexico and started inland, he feared a revolt of backsliders. So he burned his ships in the harbor. That's what your patient has to do—burn his ships behind him. Rid the house of all tobacco and smoking paraphernalia. He should announce to all his friends that he has quit smoking and specifically forbid them to "give him just one" if he weakens. Perhaps he can put some money on his ability to quit—make a bet with his wife that the smoking habit can be kicked or promise himself a trip to Florida as a reward.

Give your prospective nonsmoker one more tip. When that overwhelming urge for a cigarette strikes, tell him to hold out just *2 minutes*. By that time, the urge will have passed. Sure, it will come back; wait 2 minutes again. Every day the urge to smoke will dwindle a little.

Pulmonary function can be tested in the office or home without a spirometer. The patient who cannot blow out an ordinary paper match 12 inches in front of his mouth probably has impaired pulmonary compliance. A less flammable test uses a party noisemaker—the kind that rolls out when the horn is blown. Your patient should be able to operate this simple toy with ease; you should suspect pulmonary disorder in the patient who puffs and fails.

Postural drainage, beneficial in productive chronic bronchitis and bronchiectasis, describes the simple act of lying over the edge of a bed with the chest and head dependent (Fig. 5–1). As any schoolchild will tell you, fluids flow downhill; postural drainage allows stagnant secretions to flow from the recesses of the lungs, clearing the way for free breathing during the rest of the day.

Of course, **asthma** causes many cases of wheezing, usually associated with one or more of the following factors: family tendency, allergy, emotions, climate, and infection. I know that when I see an asthma patient in the morning, I will probably see a few more later that day; somehow, the weather conditions are right for asthma. Be wary of asthma attacks in an allergic youngster who has acquired a new cat or dog, and watch out for the youngster in the middle of a family squabble. Remember too that those "inert gases" in the spray deodorant or hair spray can may trigger an asthma attack.

Dried-out sticky secretions block the flow of air in asthma. Along with adrenalin, cortisone, aminophylline, and the other drugs you prescribe for the acute asthma attack, give the patient water, glass after glass, to restore hydration of bronchial secretions. As the adrenalin reduces bronchial spasm, the tenacious sputum comes up with coughing. What

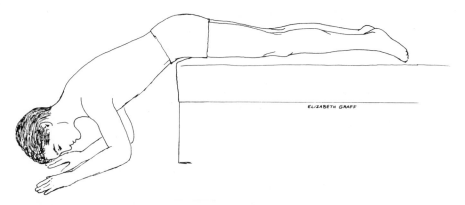

ELIZABETH GRAFF

Fig. 5–1. Postural drainage.

if the stomach becomes overdistended and the patient vomits? Good!
Emesis effectively clears bronchial secretions.

Pneumonia is a word that strikes terror to your patient's heart. Older
persons vividly remember the prayerful vigil waiting for the crisis of
pneumonia. The younger physician may hear a few râles in one lung
base, note a low-grade fever, assure the patient that he has mild pneumonia, prescribe penicillin confidently, and send the patient home. The
patient knows: He's going home to die! That's what people with pneumonia do. Doctor, please, if you are going to use the emotionally
charged word "pneumonia," be prepared to back-up your diagnosis
with x-rays and admit the patient to the hospital. But you say your
patient isn't that sick; you just hear a few rattles at one lung base. Fine,
diagnose "bronchitis" or "chest congestion," prescribe penicillin, and
dismiss the patient without scaring him to death with the word "pneumonia."

Scarlet fever, like pneumonia, is a diagnosis that terrifies older persons, who recall the scarlet fever death of Beth in *Little Women*. Carefully reassure the parents of the child with scarlet fever that the disease
is no more dangerous than any other streptococcal sore throat. Sometimes I suggest that grandparents be told *after* the child has recovered.

HEART DISEASE

Chest pain presents a diagnostic dilemma, often with life-or-death
consequences. The telephone rings at 2 A.M., and you dash out to examine a middle-aged businessman who was awakened from sleep by a

heavy gassy pain in the lower chest and epigastrium. He feels nauseous but not short of breath. The pain radiates to his right shoulder, and there are beads of perspiration on his forehead. His blood pressure is a little lower than usual and the pulse is fast. Careful auscultation of the heart reveals no abnormalities. Now what do you do with him?

It can be a lonely decision in the middle of the night. Admit him to the hospital, and the pain is sure to turn out to be simple indigestion, now complicated by a 5-day confinement and a $700 bill for hospital services. Treat him at home and he will certainly reward you by dying in bed later that night.

How about the electrocardiogram? If the patient is considerate enough to have his chest pain during office hours or if you are clever enough to lug along your electrocardiograph at 2 A.M., you can do a tracing. If there are obvious electrocardiographic signs of an acute infarction, there's your diagnosis. But don't trust the normal tracing. Many a patient with acute myocardial infarction records a textbook-normal EKG tracing only to drop his S-T segment and flip his T-waves 12 hours later.

Doctor, there's only one safe course of action with this patient: Admit him to the hospital! In fact, you will probably want to admit him to the coronary care unit and treat him as though he has an acute myocardial infarction until serial electrocardiograms and enzyme studies confirm or negate this diagnosis.

Pericarditis can present a puzzling diagnostic picture, particularly if you don't think of the disease. When your patient complains of severe chest pain and sits leaning forward from the waist to obtain relief (Fig. 5–2), you should think, "pericarditis."

Pacemakers have introduced some interesting problems to modern medicine. Pacemaker hosts should avoid electric razors, power tools, power transmission lines, and transformers—all capable of blocking pacemaker activity.

In 1937, Karel Frederik Wenckebach wrote in *Lancet:* "I owe my reputation to the fact that I use **digitalis** in doses the textbooks say are dangerous and in cases that the textbooks say are unsuitable." Yes, not all patients require exactly 0.25 mg of digoxin. For a few patients that dose is toxic; others require two or three times that amount. Titrate your digitalis dosage carefully and you will find the drug much more useful.

How about that loading dose of digitalis? Not needed, unless you are in a hurry. Most mild chronic congestive heart failure can be satisfactorily controlled by *beginning* with a maintenance dose, avoiding the nausea and vomiting that commonly accompany the "initial digitaliza-

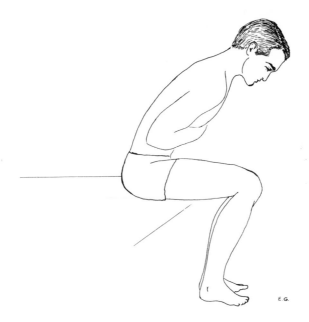

E.G.

Fig. 5–2. Pericarditis posture.

tion" procedure. Of course, in **severe** congestive heart failure and pulmonary edema, rapid digitalization is indicated, probably parenterally.

PERIPHERAL VASCULAR DISEASE

Sir William Osler wrote: "The physics of a man's circulation are the physics of the waterworks of the town in which he lives, but once out of gear, you cannot apply the same rules for the repair of the one as of the other." The analogy is a good one: Pressure rises, pressure falls, pipes corrode, weak spots leak, and obstruction blocks the flow. The plumber can shut off the water for a few hours while he works, but the doctor must keep the circulation going during repairs.

To many patients the **blood pressure** is a mystical measurement telling the doctor secrets and enabling him to diagnose a wealth of occult illnesses. Doctor, always take the blood pressure yourself. Don't relegate this important procedure to a nurse.

High blood pressure readings are readily obtained on a patient rushed into the examination room after a 2-hour wait reviewing old magazines, ordered to undress by a cheerless aide, then assaulted by the physician who begins the interview by choking the upper arm with his blood pressure cuff. Remember that blood pressure varies 10 to 20 mm Hg from minute to minute. Let your patient sit down, catch his breath, get used to the room, and talk a little before you measure his blood pressure. Your reading will be much more reliable. Think you have an artificially high reading? Don't be afraid to take the pressure again at the end of the examination.

How to determine the blood pressure of Mrs. Adiposity, whose upper arms are the size of a line-backer's thighs? Move the blood pressure cuff down to her forearm and place the stethoscope head over the radial artery.

While we're talking about Mrs. Adiposity, do you know how to weigh her? Once she stepped on your 300-lb-maximum-weight office scales and the little weights all went "clunk" in protest. Use two ordinary bathroom scales. Place one of the patient's delicate feet on each scale and add the total. The sum will be accurate within a pound or two, and when you weigh more than 300 lb, that's pretty accurate.

Arterial occlusion may develop gradually or abruptly. The sudden cold painful foot is a surgical emergency, requiring prompt diagnosis and bold therapy. More commonly, the patient with occlusive arterial disease comes to the office with a history of pain in the legs. Careful questioning may reveal the typical story of intermittent claudication— the predictable occurrence of aching leg pain after walking a certain distance. Your senior citizen patient describes how he stops to look in every fifth store window to rest his legs.

Check the dorsalis pedis artery. Have trouble finding it in older persons with impaired circulation? Remember, the dorsalis pedis artery forms an equilateral triangle with the medial and lateral malleoli (Fig. 5–3).

Sure there is no dorsalis pedis artery palpable? Then check the posterior tibial artery, found where the name describes. Not there? Then move up the leg, checking the popliteal and femoral pulses. Here's a clue: The claudication pain is usually located about 6 inches below the arterial obstruction.

Think one foot is cooler than the other? Use the back of your hand to compare; it is much more sensitive to temperature changes than the palm or fingertips. Move your hands back and forth from one foot to the other and you should be able to detect minor temperature variations.

Your office should have an oscillometer, to measure arterial blood flow to the extremities. A good oscillometer costs about $70 and will last

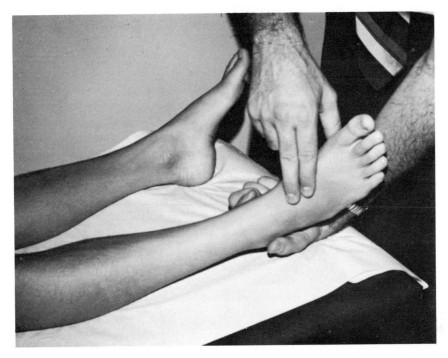

Fig. 5–3. The dorsalis pedis triangle.

until you cash in your retirement fund. You may use this expensive toy only four or five times a year, but when indicated, there is no substitute for the oscillometer in the diagnosis of occlusive arterial disease.

Venous varicosities of the lower extremities, the curse of the patient's ancestors, usually receive several years of medical therapy before falling prey to the surgeon. There is no more useful therapy for venous varicosities than the Jobst elastic stockings. But, having spent the patient's time and money on these fine custom-made surgical hose, have you told him how to put them on? The patient should don his elastic surgical hose in the morning before he arises from bed. This helps prevent the venous distention that occurs upon assuming the upright position.

Here's a tip: The rocking chair promotes arterial perfusion and venous return in the lower extremities. Popularized by Dr. Janet Travell while she was personal physician to President John F. Kennedy, the rocking chair can help prevent thrombophlebitis and consequent pulmonary embolism following medical illness and surgical procedures.

DISEASES OF THE GASTROINTESTINAL TRACT

Hiccups can test the equanimity of your most placid patient, interfering with eating, sleeping, and breathing. There is no single sure-fire cure for hiccups, but they may respond to one or another of the following measures:

1. Rebreathing carbon dioxide from a paper bag held over the face
2. Drinking a glass of water holding a pencil clenched in the teeth
3. Passing a nasogastric tube and aspirating the stomach contents
4. Inhaling whiffs of ether
5. Injecting diazepam (Valium), 5 to 10 mg intramuscularly
6. Injecting atropine sulfate, 0.5 to 1 mg subcutaneously
7. Administering 10% calcium gluconate solution, 10 ml intravenously

Nasogastric tube placement can be difficult. Is the tip in the stomach or coiled around the nasopharynx pointing down the larynx? Before starting tube feeding or injecting 50 ml of saline, find out where the tip of the nasogastric tube lies. Place a stethoscope over the patient's stomach, withdraw the plunger of an empty 10- or 20-ml syringe, place the syringe in the exposed end of the nasogastric tube, and sharply close the plunger, forcing air down the tube. If the tube is correctly placed, a reassuring bubbling sound will be heard in the stomach.

The **string test for upper gastrointestinal bleeding** helps localize the bleeding site. When you are not sure exactly where the source of upper gastrointestinal bleeding lies, have the patient swallow one end of a 36-inch length of string after you have carefully measured the apparent distance between his nose and stomach. Leave the string in place a few minutes, then withdraw it. The bleeding site will usually show clearly as a blood-stained segment of the string, beginning abruptly, with some staining below, as blood passes through the stomach. The string test will often localize bleeding when x-rays fail.

Here are two diagnostic tips. File them away in the recesses of your memory. Some day one of them may be important:

1. Indigestion for meat is an early symptom of cancer of the stomach.
2. The patient repeatedly awakened from sleep by crampy abdominal pain has cancer of the bowel until proved otherwise.

Constipation, celebrated in TV commercials, is a common complaint of older patients. Watch out for antispasmodics, codeine, and iron; they constipate. Encourage your constipated patient to drink six full glasses of water a day. Some of my elderly patients tell me that a glass of hot water flavored with lemon taken in the morning assures a normal bowel movement that day. Bran flakes and prune juice are good physiologic stimulants, and don't forget the beneficial effect of one to three daily teaspoonsful of psyllium hydrophilic mucilloid (Metamucil).

Fecal impaction is the penalty for poor bowel hygiene. Although sometimes noted following barium x-ray examination, fecal impaction usually occurs in inactive older persons with marginal consumption of roughage and water. The Fleet brand oil enema helps in the removal of a fecal impaction. Keep a few of these disposable enemas in your office. A plastic bedpan (fracture type) is also a help in the office removal of a fecal impaction.

When a house-call patient with severe abdominal pain turns out to have a fecal impaction, you will be glad you carry a disposable rectal glove, a small single-dose envelope of Lubafax surgical lubricant, and paper towels in your house-call bag.

THE SKIN AS A MIRROR OF DISEASE

In the early nineteenth century, François Magendie wrote: "Medicine is a science in the making." In 1971, we took another small step along the road from witchcraft to science, with the introduction of phototherapy for infections due to the **herpes simplex** virus. The early vesicles are ruptured with a sterile needle and painted with 0.1% aqueous solution of proflavine or neutral red dye. After 5 minutes, the lesions are exposed to a 15-watt daylight-type fluorescent light for 15 minutes at a distance of 6 inches. The therapy is repeated 1 to 4 hours later and on subsequent days as necessary. Excellent results and good patient acceptance result in most cases.

Jaundice may be noted on the skin before conjunctival discoloration is noted. Experienced nurses don't look for jaundice in a newborn baby's eyes: They blanche a spot on his forehead with finger pressure to detect icterus. In your older patients, check untanned skin of the abdomen for early evidence of jaundice.

Petechiae indicate capillary bleeding, associated with a bewildering number of infectious, hematologic, and degenerative conditions. Is that skin lesion a rash or petechiae? A rash blanches on pressure; petechiae don't blanch.

How about that youngster with fever, lethargy, sore throat, and petechiae? Of course, you will think of meningitis, but don't forget that streptococcal infections can cause petechiae too.

Do you remember how to test for capillary fragility? On the patient's forearm, draw a circle 2.5 cm in diameter (a two-bit piece is the right size). Apply the blood pressure cuff at 50 mm pressure for 15 minutes, then remove the cuff and examine the circle 2 minutes later (Fig. 5–4). More than 20 petechiae is definitely abnormal.

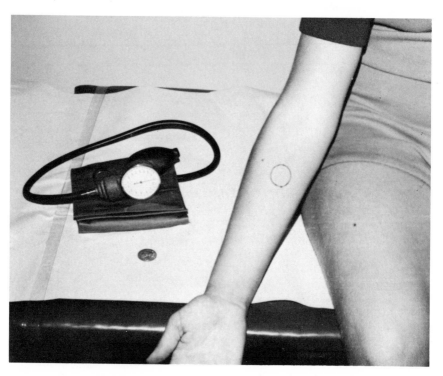

Fig. 5–4. The capillary fragility test.

Hypersensitivity plagues the unwary skin. How many times have you cured impetigo to leave the patient with a neomycin hypersensitivity dermatitis? Are those "caine" sunburn preparations going to lead to local anesthetic reactions in years to come?

Parabens are highly sensitizing preservatives found in many topical steroid creams, occasionally aggravating the contact rash. Betamethasone valerate (Valisone) cream contains no parabens.

Follow this rule: Don't use on the skin any medication that the patient might later receive internally.

The danger of **photosensitization** is familiar to the modern physician, but be especially wary of prescribing demeclocycline (Declomycin) during summer months. Experience has shown that Declomycin can cause an exaggerated sunburn response—more commonly and more pronounced than other tetracyclines.

DISEASES OF THE NERVOUS SYSTEM

God may forgive you your sins, but your nervous system won't.

Alfred Korzybski
(1879–1950)

The **patellar reflex,** all-important in the neurologic examination and assessment of the thyroid status, may exhibit all the vigor of a wet noodle. Is the reflex really absent? Enhance the patellar deep tendon reflex by forced plantar flexion of the great toe, instructing the patient to push his large toe down against your finger (Fig. 5–5).

The **tuning fork,** like the oscillometer, lies idle most of the time, but when you test for diabetic neuropathy or posterolateral sclerosis, there is no substitute. Use your tuning fork on healthy patients to learn the normal response.

Two-point discrimination can be tested with the same calipers you use to read your electrocardiograms. Measure the distances between the points on any millimeter ruler. You don't have an EKG caliper? Then purchase a 10-cent comb with teeth 2 mm apart. Break off teeth to leave spaces 2, 4, 6, 8, and 10 mm between remaining teeth and you have an accurate instrument for determining two-point discrimination.

Testing **cold perception** is easy. Use the cold chrome part of your reflex hammer. Or you can use test tubes filled with hot and cold water from the tap in your examination room.

Facial weakness can mean Bell's palsy or a stroke on the involved side. Can you tell the difference? Keep this in mind. The stroke victim, who has intact nerve centers on the other hemisphere, can partially wrinkle his forehead by looking up at the ceiling. The patient with Bell's

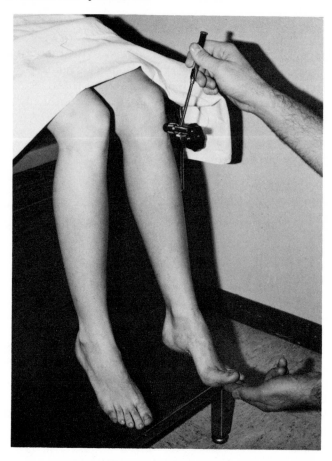

Fig. 5–5. Forced plantar flexion of the great toe enhances the patellar reflex.

palsy, which involves the peripheral nerves, cannot wrinkle his forehead.

Tremor of the hands can be subtle, especially the fine tremor of hyperthyroidism. Dramatize that tremor by placing an ordinary sheet of paper on the back of the patient's outstretched hand. A fine tremor will flutter that paper like leaves in an autumn wind.

The **caffeine-withdrawal headache** could be mentioned in the next chapter on surgery, because the surgeon and anesthesiologist often face the dilemma. Middle-aged Mrs. Jones enters the hospital feeling well for an elective surgical procedure. The morning after her operation, she complains bitterly of a severe aching frontal headache, unresponsive to simple analgesia. What's the answer? Mrs. Jones is suffering withdrawal symptoms; she misses her eight cups of coffee a day. The caffeine-withdrawal headache can be treated with oxygen, 500 mg of caffeine sodium benzoate intramuscularly, or, almost too simple, a cup of coffee.

The **hangover headache,** the penalty for overindulgence the night before, seems determined to explode the cranium. Along with analgesics and fatherly advice, try whiffs of oxygen and the intramuscular injection of 2 ml of B complex vitamins.

Hypochondriasis eludes classification within organ systems. Usually armed with a long list of multiple complaints, the hypochondriac settles down to a detailed discussion of each carefully tabulated ache and pain. Don't dismiss him lightly, and don't neglect to examine every area of complaint. Hypochondriacs get sick too. Remember, somewhere in all that rhetoric may be the first symptom of serious illness.

References and Suggestions for Further Reading

1. Ayres S M, Gianelli S Jr: Care of the Critically Ill. New York, Appleton, 1967.
2. Ayres S M, Gregory J J, Buehler M E: Cardiology: A Clinicophysiologic Approach. New York, Appleton, 1971.
3. Bartel A, Tyroler H A, Heyden S: Electrocardiographic predictors of coronary heart disease. Arch Intern Med 128:929–937, 1971.
4. Beetham W P: Physical Examination of the Joints. Philadelphia, Saunders, 1970.
5. Conklin E F: Use of permanent transvenous pacemaker in 168 consecutive patients. Am Heart J 82:4–14, 1971.
6. Duggan J J, Schiess W A, Hilfinger M F Jr: Unheeded signals of fatal coronary artery disease. N Y State J Med 71:2639–2642, 1971.
7. Duke M: Bed rest in acute myocardial infarction: Study of physician practices. Am Heart J 82:486–491; 1971.
8. Fowler N O: Cardiac Diagnosis. New York, Harper & Row, 1968.
9. Hinshaw H C, Garland L H: Diseases of the Chest. Philadelphia, Saunders, 1969.
10. Kirby W M M: Modern management of respiratory diseases. Med Clin North 51:-269–578, 1967.
11. Leibowitz J O: The History of Coronary Heart Disease. Berkeley, Calif, University of California Press, 1970.
12. Schuster M M: Functional gastrointestinal disorders. GP 35:131–139, 1967.
13. Singer H C: Familial aspects of inflammatory bowel disease. Gastroenterology 61:-423–430, 1971.
14. Weinblatt E, Shapiro S, Frank C W: Changes in personal characteristics of men, over five years, following first diagnosis of coronary heart disease. Am J Public Health 61:831–842, 1971.
15. Wenckebach K F: Principle of easing load. Ned Tijdschr Geneeskd 81:367–372, 1937.

6

Sensible Surgery

A chirurgien should have three dyvers properties in his person. That is to saie, a harte as the harte of a lyon, his eyes like the eyes of a hawke, and his handes the handes of a woman.

John Halle (1529–1568)
Epistle to the Reader in his trans-
lation of Lanfranc's Chirurgia
Parva

Office surgery offers the physician a wide range of self-expression, whether tying off skin tags or the cosmetic repair of extensive lacerations. A minimum of equipment is necessary, practice is essential, and a knowledge of possible complications is mandatory. Don't start anything you can't finish. Temper your scalpel with cool common sense and enjoy this integral part of the office practice of medicine.

There is one hospital surgical dictum you should remember. Take your time closing the skin; it's the only part of the operation the patient sees. You may have spent an hour repairing delicate subcutaneous structures, but if the scar looks sloppy, the patient looks askance at the surgeon.

OFFICE PROCEDURES

Surgical sterility worries many potential office surgeons. Certainly, your treatment room is no place to remove a gallbladder; but, because the skin can repel a host of invading bacteria, ritual operating room sterility is not required for office surgery.

Sir William Osler wrote: "Soap and water and common sense are the best disinfectants." Scrub the wound and your hands with plenty of soap and water; rinse copiously. The surgical gown and mask are not necessary. Many office surgeons operate bare-handed, but I prefer to use sterile gloves. A good quality "disposable" surgical glove can be scrubbed, autoclaved, and reused over and over.

Keep your treatment room "clean." Infected wounds should be relegated to an examination room, and the treatment room reserved for surgical therapy of uninfected lesions.

How much sterility is needed? The **thrombosed external hemorrhoid** responds well to evacuation through a 1 cm radial incision following the intraepidermal infiltration of 1 ml of 2% lidocaine (Xylocaine). Not a chance of keeping this wound clean. Disposable examination gloves protect the surgeon's hands as well as sterile surgical gloves, and dressings should be clean but need not be autoclaved.

Skin tags are easy to remove. An internist friend tells me this is the only surgical procedure he does. A silk thread is tied tightly around the base of the tag, obliterating its blood supply. Within a week or two, the skin tag falls off. Multiple skin tags respond to light electrocautery. No anesthesia is required for patients with a normal pain threshold, and 50 or more skin tags can be removed at one session.

Here's a tip about electrocautery that you should learn from a book rather than by personal experience: Don't use alcohol or ethyl chloride on the skin prior to electrical cautery. Flash burns can result!

Keloids can occur in spite of your best surgical efforts and may be rightfully blamed on the individual patient's healing mechanism. Excise the keloid at your peril; another is likely to form. Some keloids respond to the intralesional injection of 25 mg. of triamcinolone diacetate (Aristocort Intralesional), followed by the topical application of 0.1% Aristocort cream. Those keloids that fail to respond should be treated expectantly or referred to a plastic surgeon.

Foreign bodies under the skin look easy to remove. You can palpate a pellet of buckshot, and a piece of pencil lead looks as big as a cannonball. But as soon as you make your incision in the skin, they submerge in a welter of blood and fat. Plan your foreign body removal attempt carefully; get x-rays, including multiple views with skin markers. Don't attempt the procedure without proper instruments and plenty of time. Can't find that steel fragment? Leave the wound open, instructing the patient to soak it in warm salt water for 30 minutes four times daily, and try again 2 or 3 days later. Still can't find it? Let your incision heal. Many veterans still carry shrapnel fragments from World War II; that tiny foreign body will probably never cause your patient any trouble.

Ganglion of the wrist causes more concern than pain. Most should be treated with reassurance, but a few enlarge and cause pain, prompting operative intervention. Many ganglia can be aspirated with a 15-gauge needle under local anesthesia. Following aspiration, apply a tight compression bandage to be left in place for 5 days. Although aspiration is sometimes curative, many ganglia recur, and if further surgery is warranted, the patient should be referred to a specialist.

Plantar wart therapy fills volumes. Witchcraft, hypnosis, and ritual scrubbing have all been tried. Surgical excision is, of course, effective, at the price of short-term disability. Electrocautery may result in painful plantar scarring, as much trouble to the patient as the wart. Ultrasound treatments have been recommended, but ultrasound should be used cautiously over growing bones and, unfortunately, most plantar warts occur in schoolage children.

Bichloroacetic acid therapy is effective against plantar warts, and produces minimal discomfort and no disability. At 2-week intervals, bichloroacetic acid is applied to the wart and covered with nonporous adhesive tape for a few hours after treatment. No change in the patient's activities is required, other than the admonition not to infect others by walking barefoot at home or in the locker room at school. At each subsequent visit, the core is carefully removed with a spoon curette, and the next layer is cauterized with acid. Most plantar warts disappear following four to six treatments.

Ear piercing, like tattooing, is a permanent cosmetic procedure. When a schoolgirl asks to have her ears pierced, I always recall a cartoon I once saw of an austere matron in evening dress at the opera; on her deltoid was tattooed, "Win with Willkie." Ear piercing can lead to infections and keloids, but if your patient is determined, the doctor will do a better job than her teenage friends.

Locate the spot on each ear with a skin-marking pen. Don't pierce too low; her earlobes will sag as she gets older. Then stand back and see if the two ears match. After injecting a minimal amount of Xylocaine, pierce the earlobe with an 18-gauge needle and insert the gold posts. Instruct your patient to rotate the posts daily, but not to remove them until the tract has epithelialized—usually about a month. Pierced ears don't tolerate cheap nickel earrings; advise your ear-pierced ladies to wear only bona fide gold earrings.

SURGICAL DIAGNOSIS

The office examination of the potentially surgical problem can be as important as the operation itself, particularly if the examining physician misses the diagnosis.

An **infant's hernia** may be reported by his mother. "Every time Johnny cries, he gets this lump in his groin." But, of course, when Johnny comes to the office, no hernia can be found. How to get Johnny to increase his intraabdominal pressure? Tickle his ribs until he laughs. Try examining his ears and throat; most infants will begin crying, popping out the hernia. Have the older child stand and blow up a balloon to demonstrate the elusive hernia.

The **ventral hernia** or diastasis recti abdominis in an adult is demonstrated by having the supine patient lift his head to look at his toes. Still can't find it? Then examine the patient standing, holding his breath and straining.

Appendicitis virtually always prompts a call to the doctor. An occasional case of vomiting can safely be treated with fluids, but all children or adults whose overriding complaint is abdominal pain should be examined promptly. Here are two tips to aid the diagnosis of appendicitis: Rarely is the appendicitis patient hungry and he has almost always skipped the last meal. The latter is an important diagnostic point and a boon to the anesthesiologist. The physical examination of the suspected appendicitis victim is incomplete without a rectal examination. The retrocecal appendix, hiding under folds of mesentery, can sometimes be detected only upon rectal examination.

Adhesions do occur, but make that diagnosis reluctantly, only after thorough examination and testing to exclude other causes of abdominal distress. Too often, patients accept the diagnosis of adhesions only to later develop clear symptoms of regional enteritis or carcinoma of the pancreas. As Osler said: "Adhesions are the refuge of the diagnostically destitute."

Sigmoidoscopy is a necessary evil. Did you ever stop and think, "What is the patient worried about while I have this long silver tube in his rectum?" I'll tell you! He's worried that he will defecate all over the table and the doctor. Reassure him that, while the sigmoidoscope is in place, bowel movement is impossible.

Be careful with that air during sigmoidoscopy. Distention of the bowel hurts! And be sure to let the air out before removing the sigmoidoscope or your patient will be socially unacceptable for the next hour.

LACERATIONS

Most simple lacerations can be repaired in the office, sparing your patient a trip to the hospital and the obligatory emergency room fee. Your **instruments** should be packed in a suture set, sealed and autoclaved, ready for instant use. Because lacerations do not occur by appointment, your office should have several identical suture sets, including these instruments:

1. Combination needle holder and scissors
2. Sharp iris scissors
3. Adson forceps with teeth
4. Small hemostat
5. Sterile drapes (I use autoclaved professional paper towels)
6. Cotton-tipped applicators
7. Medicine cup to hold water, Zephiran, etc.
8. A stack of autoclaved 4-inch by 4-inch gauze pads

The **suture material** is chosen according to the extent and location of the laceration. Delicate 5–0 suture material is indicated in facial lacerations; heavier 3–0 sutures should be used in larger lacerations on the extremities. While black silk remains an acceptable skin suture material, I prefer the synthetic fibers that will stretch to accommodate swelling, then return to their original length. Ethilon monofilament nylon with a cutting needle is a good choice for most minor surgical repairs.

The **type of stitch** influences the final repair. The intern's stitch (through and through, tie, and be damned) is still the most widely used and is acceptable for most wound repairs.

The mattress stitch takes a little longer, but distributes tension over a wider area of skin and allows better apposition of skin edges; use the mattress repair in large lacerations over joints and in areas with tension on the suture line.

The subcuticular repair makes a neat closure, suture removal is unnecessary and the patient is pleased—unless foreign body reactions cause stitch abscesses along the line of repair.

The running lock repair is occasionally used on lacerations, but a single break in the suture material can lead to a widely gaping wound.

Remember that the skin treats suture material as a foreign body. Use only enough sutures to close the wound neatly. Don't pull them too tight. And promptly remove any individual suture showing evidence of a stitch abscess.

Restraining the uncooperative child takes technique, not strength. Mummy the youngster in a sheet only as a last resort. How much more reassuring to have the nurse or mother sit at the head of the table, confidently holding the child's extended arms locked securely against his head (Fig. 6–1). If the child is really unruly, a second helper can hold his feet. Pick mother rather than father as helper. When Shakespeare wrote, "Many will swoon when they do look on blood," he meant fathers. As a rule, mothers are much better equipped emotionally to assist your surgical repair.

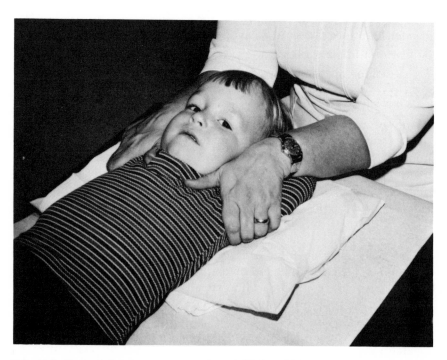

Fig. 6–1. Restraining an uncooperative child for office surgery.

Prepare the area carefully, removing excess hair. A recent study compared the results of hair removal by depilatory and by shaving in a series of surgical patients. The razor-shaved patients had 10 times as many postoperative infections as the depilatory-treated patients.

Scalp lacerations, however, require careful preparation with scissors and razor shaving. Take your time. Careful preparation is the most important aspect of scalp laceration repairs. Don't be tempted to leave the hair in place and suture through it; a week later you will find yourself rummaging for suture ends in a clotted, infected mass of hair and dried blood.

When shaving the scalp wound, think about the final dressing. I use rectangular Elastoplast bandages on small scalp wounds; these require a rectangular surgical field so the dressing does not end up in the hair.

Jagged dirty lacerations leave ragged ugly scars unless converted to sharp linear lacerations by careful debridement. Use your scalpel on a jagged laceration before reaching for your suture. Flush copiously; there may be dirt particles trapped inside. Examine the wound with the loupe; you may be surprised to find how much foreign material is left.

Flap lacerations leave cosmetically unattractive scars as the upper segment of the flap retracts, forming scar tissue. Careful debridement helps convert the flap to a linear laceration with sides perpendicular to the skin (Fig. 6–2), allowing a physiologic repair with less postoperative scarring.

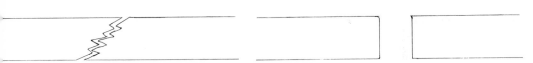

Fig. 6–2. Convert a flap laceration (left) to a linear laceration (right) for a more cosmetically acceptable repair.

Tongue lacerations require repair only if a flap is hanging loose (Fig. 6–3). Tack the flap back to the body of the tongue with a single heavy black silk suture, placed without anesthesia if the patient is cooperative. Linear lacerations of the body of the tongue heal spontaneously without suturing.

In 1912, William Stewart Halsted wrote in the *Bulletin of the Johns Hopkins Hospital:* "The only weapon with which the unconscious pa-

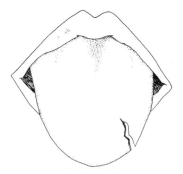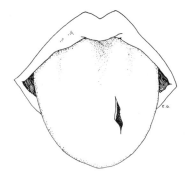

Fig. 6–3. Repair a tongue laceration if a flap is hanging loose (left), but not if the tear is in the body of the tongue (right).

tient can immediately retaliate upon the incompetent surgeon is hemorrhage." That **deep laceration** pumping blood is a problem. If your sponge-clamp-and-tie efforts are unsuccessful, try placing a wide suture around the bleeding area, tied tightly. The blood flow will usually cease promptly, and you can get on with your repair.

A **hematoma** under your laceration repair delays healing and invites infection. It is better prevented that treated. Obliterate subcutaneous pockets with chromic catgut sutures. Use pressure dressings whenever indicated, and inspect suspicious wounds frequently. If in doubt, leave an autoclaved ordinary rubber band in the wound as a drain and remove it 2 or 3 days later as the danger of hematoma formation passes.

POSTOPERATIVE WOUND CARE

In the sixteenth century Ambroise Paré said: "I dressed him and God healed him." But the best surgical efforts of God and man have been foiled by inappropriate postoperative care.

The dressing on most simple lacerations should be changed daily—more often if wet or dirty. Instruct the patient not to wash away the healing scab. Splints should be used when lacerations occur on the extensor skin over joints, and an Ace bandage can reinforce the dressing over difficult-to-bandage areas. Tincture of benzoin helps hold tape on sweaty skin after minor surgery.

Scalp wounds receive a festive array of dressings—most inappropriate or unnecessary. If carefully shaved to accommodate the final dressing, large scalp wounds can be dressed with a Telfa pad cut to fit the wound and held in place with Elastoplast tape glued down with tincture of benzoin. This dressing will stay in place for 7 to 10 days unless purposely picked off by inquisitive fingers. By suture removal time, hair bristles have elevated the dressing, making removal easy. If still stuck tight, alcohol is an excellent solvent for tincture of benzoin. Sure, scalp dressings take a little time, but don't repair a scalp laceration and spray it with a sticky transparent glop. That is not a dressing.

Suture removal must be carefully timed, balancing the possibility of wound separation against the likelihood of a foreign body reaction. In general, sutures in the face are removed at about 5 days, although some more adventuresome surgeons will argue for less. Sutures on the body, arms, and upper legs are removed at 1 week; those on the hands, knees, feet, and ankles are often best left in place for 10 to 14 days.

When removing sutures, form the habit of taking out alternate stitches and evaluating the closure before proceeding. Many times the first hint of separation will be noted, and the remaining sutures can be left in place another 3 or 4 days.

Stitch abscesses are the body's reaction to a foreign substance, more likely to occur the longer sutures are in place. If a stitch abscess occurs, remove the offending suture (Fig. 6–4), but don't pull the infected end through the suture tract. Stitch abscesses in subcutaneous sutures are best left undisturbed until they pop through the surface. Warm soaks will speed the process, but suppress the urge to open the wound. The body will extrude these sutures in good time.

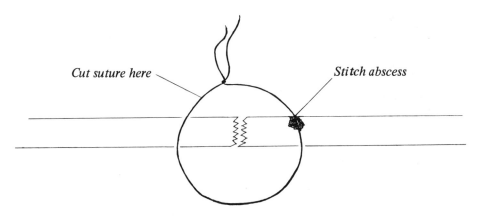

Fig. 6–4. Correct method of removing an infected suture.

The **abdominal binder** is a fine old medical instrument that has fallen into disuse in our rush to graft arteries and transplant hearts. Don't forget its value in the overweight patient following abdominal surgery, particularly when a midline incision was necessary. You may have to show a young nurse how it is properly applied, starting at the bottom, flap over flap, until a single safety pin at the top holds the binder in place.

SURGERY OF THE NAILS

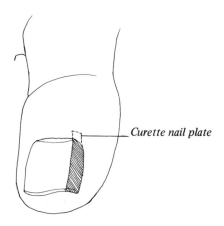

Curette nail plate

Fig. 6–5. Correction of an ingrown toenail by excision of part of the nail.

Ingrown toenails arise from a variety of vices, including cutting rounded corners, wearing tight shoes, and overeating to the point of obesity so that flabby skin margins are pushed up around the nail by the body weight. Many ingrown toenails can be prevented by cutting the toenails straight across, wearing properly fitted shoes, and losing weight. Also try this simple device: Wedge a wad of cotton under the partially ingrown nail corner and hold it in place with flexible collodion as a glue. Ordinary household cement works almost as well. The glued-in wad of cotton will stay in place for several weeks, depressing the skin margin and elevating the nail.

The short-term surgical correction of an ingrown toenail is easy; the biggest problem is providing adequate anesthesia. Regional anesthesia should be attained by injecting 1 ml of 2% Xylocaine adjacent to the digital nerves at the base of the great toe. Then wait patiently for 5 to

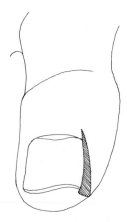

Fig. 6–6. Correction of an ingrown toenail by removal of a flap of skin.

7 minutes until anesthesia is complete. Elevate the offending nail margin all the way to the base, a width of about ¼ inch. A heavy silver probe works well. Use sturdy scissors to cut the ¼-inch nail margin free, again all the way to the base, then curette the nail plate thoroughly (Fig. 6–5). A sterile dressing completes the procedure, and the patient is discharged with instructions to soak the toe in warm salt water for 30 minutes three times daily until the exposed nail bed is dry. Although this will correct some cases of ingrown toenail, many will recur and require the more extensive definitive procedure described next.

Using the above-described digital nerve block on the great toe, leave the nail undisturbed and remove the tissue flap by means of a pie-shaped incision, closed with Steri-Strips. (Fig. 6–6). Postoperative soaking is not indicated and the Steri-Strips are removed in about 10 days. Relief of the ingrown toenail is usually long-lasting.

Evacuation of the **subungal hematoma** can be neatly performed with a hot paperclip. In fact, I haven't used my fancy $9 nail drill in years; a drilled hole seems to close over promptly, but a hole made with a hot paperclip stays open to drain. Don't use an alcohol burner to heat the clip; as the alcohol evaporates, it sputters and fumes, and the terrified victim cries. Equip your office with a simple butane cigarette lighter— the kind that stays on without being held open (Fig. 6–7).

Splinters under the nail should be easy to remove with splinter forceps unless, as usually happens, the patient and his family have tried already, broken off any accessible pieces, and driven the remaining fragment deeper into the nail bed. Instead of elevating the entire nail, try shaving through the nail with a No. 15 scalpel blade (Fig. 6–8).

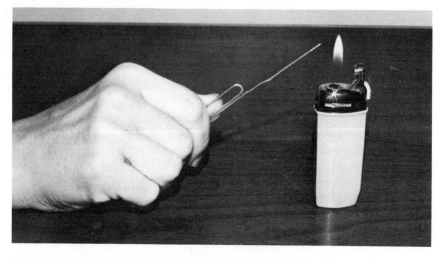

Fig. 6–7. Equipment for evacuation of a subungual hematoma.

Anesthesia is usually not necessary, and shaving down avoids separating the nail from its vascular supply in the nail bed.

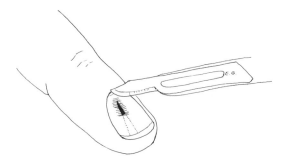

Fig. 6–8. Shaving through the nail with a scalpel blade allows removal of a broken splinter from beneath the nail.

FISHHOOKS, RINGS, AND OTHER PROBLEMS

Abrasions are painful. The child who falls from his bicycle onto gravel has more pain than the child with a laceration. And every speck of gravel must be carefully removed—a tender, time-consuming procedure. Use your loupe and plenty of light. Don't hesitate to infiltrate 1%

Xylocaine under the abrasion if extensive cleansing is necessary. Use lots of soap and water, paint with Betadine, then leave the area exposed. Abrasions heal much faster open than closed. Discourage the mother from using Vaseline and first-aid cream.

Burns require a second look. The mildly red but painful area today may be covered with blisters tomorrow. When presented with a first or possibly second degree burn, wash the area gently with Zephiran, air-dry, and cover with a Furacin gauze dressing. Reexamine in 2 or 3 days. If no blisters have developed, the burn was first degree and should be left open at this time. If vesicles have developed, some debridement will be needed, and repeated dressing changes are in order. I check, debride, and redress burns every third day until they are healed.

Watch those electrical burns. The tissue is cooked like a fried egg. The burn may not appear serious at first, but the fried tissue will deteriorate over the next few days, showing how much damage was really done.

Slicer injuries bleed and bleed. The rotary meat slicer neatly trims off a flap of skin exposing the underlying capillaries that bleed through dressing after dressing, day after day. How to stop the bleeding? Anchor a small piece of Gelfoam (the dental size is about right) tightly against the bleeding area with Steri-Strips and cover with a thick dressing (Fig. 6-9). The Gelfoam–Steri-Strip dressing should be left in place for at least a week, allowing healing to begin.

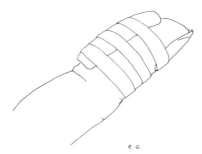

Fig. 6–9. Gelfoam–Steri-Strip therapy of a finger injured by a slicer.

A ring on a swollen finger should be removed before it begins to act as a tourniquet. But I haven't sawed through a ring in years. There is an easier way: Begin with a 36-inch length of firm string, passed under the ring, then wrapped carefully around the length of the finger. Anchor the distal end, then carefully pull the end that was passed under the ring (Fig. 6-10). In most cases, the ring will spin neatly right off the finger.

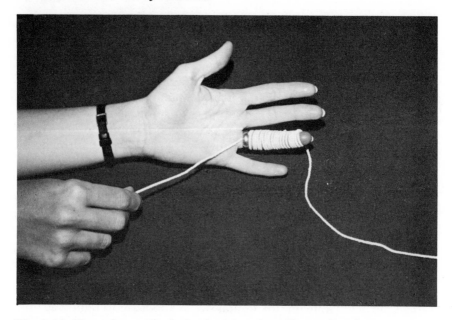

Fig. 6–10. The string method of spinning a ring off a swollen finger.

Fishhooks seek out little boys. The proper method of fishhook removal varies with the type of hook, the location, and the instruments available. Most fishhooks can be removed easily by infiltrating the area with 1 ml of 2% Xylocaine, passing the needle down the fishhook tract. Small three-point hooks are then grasped with a Kelly clamp and removed back through the tract; the barb causes little tissue damage. Large single hooks with big barbs are often best passed on through the skin, under local anesthesia, and the barbed tip removed with wire cutters or your otherwise unused ring cutter. Then the stump of the hook can be pulled back through the tract. We'll talk about the fisherman's method of hook removal in Chapter 12.

Speaking of fishing, the Kelly clamp is the world's best instrument for removing hooks from fish and may spare you the embarrassment of having a fishhook removed from your own finger.

References and Suggestions for Further Reading

1.   Alexander J W, Kaplan J Z, Altemeier W A: Role of suture materials in the development of wound infection. Ann Surg 165: 192–199, 1967.

2.   Artz C P, MacMillan B D: Treatment of burns of difficult areas. Am J Surg 91:-517–522, 1956.

3. Ballinger W F III, Rutherford R B, Zuidema G D: The Management of Trauma. Philadelphia, Saunders, 1968.

4. David L: Christopher's Textbook of Surgery, 9th ed. Philadelphia, Saunders, 1968.

5. Easson C E, Russell H M: The Curability of Cancer in Various Sites. Baltimore, Williams & Wilkins, 1968.

6. Giannestros N J: Foot Disorders: Medical and Surgical Management. Philadelphia, Lea & Febiger, 1967.

7. Gibbs R C: Calluses, corns and warts. Am Fam Physician G P 3:92–101, 1971.

8. Holgersen L O, Stanley-Brown E G: Acute appendicitis with perforation. Am J Dis Child 122:288–293, 1971.

9. Kopell H P, Winokur J, Thompson W A L: Ingrown toenail: New concept. NY State J Med 67:1215–1219, 1966.

10. Levine M: Surgical Malpractice: Surgical Errors and Accidents and Professional Liability to the Injured. Washington, D C, Trial Lawyers Service, 1970.

11. Lilly H A, Lowbury E J L: Disinfection of skin: Assessment of some new preparations. Br Med J 3:674–676, 1971.

12. Lynch J B, Wisner H K, Lewis S R: Management of electrical injuries. South Med J 64:97–103, 1971.

13. Nardi G, Zuidema G: Surgery: A Concise Guide to Clinical Practice, 2nd ed. Boston, Little Brown, 1965.

14. Raffensperger J G, Seeler R A, Moncada R: The Acute Abdomen in Infancy and Childhood. Philadelphia, Lippincott, 1970.

15. Seropain R, Reynolds B M: Wound infections after preoperative depilatory vs. razor preparation. Am J Surg 161:251–256, 1971.

16. Shires G T: Care of the Trauma Patient. New York, McGraw-Hill, 1966.

17. Smith E I: Burns in children. Postgrad Med 47:203–209, 1970.

7

The Perils of Orthopedics

"Mr. Abernethy," said a patient, "I have something the matter, Sir, with this arm. There, oh! (making a particular motion with the limb), that, Sir, gives me great pain." "Well, what a fool you must be to do it, then," said Abernethy.

John Abernethy
(1764–1831)
Quoted by George Macilwain

Orthopedics, the science of sprains, pains, bends, and breaks, is, indeed, a physical discipline. Physical principles, including leverage, fulcrums, and force arms, meld with materia medica. Injuries occur as suddenly and as unexpectedly as an automobile accident, often requiring decisive therapeutic action. Pitfalls are everywhere, and a misstep can result in deformity and prolonged disability. The orthopedic surgeon boasts the dubious distinction of higher professional liability insurance rates than most other specialties, attesting to the perils of his calling.

THE ORTHOPEDIC EXAMINATION

The bony skeleton and the forces that move it are the province of orthopedics. Your examination begins the minute you lay eyes on the patient, watching the way he walks, stands, and sits. Watch his eyes for evidence of pain upon movement. Does your patient sit comfortably or stand during the interview? Does the man seeking compensation for a back injury remove his coat and shirt with difficulty? Or does he lithely strip off his clothing and hop to your examination table like a young gazelle?

Leonardo da Vinci observed: "No muscle uses its power in pushing but always in drawing to itself the parts that are joined to it." Think about the muscles, joints, and bones involved. Name them. What is their function? How did the injury occur? Do the physical findings corroborate the patient's history? What complications might be expected?

Roentgenography is an integral part of the orthopedic examination, omitted seldom, and then at your peril. Unless handy to a hospital x-ray department, the physician encountering a number of orthopedic and industrial injuries should have x-ray facilities in the office. (The office x-ray unit is discussed in Chapter 18.) Two views are minimum; three are better. In all youngsters and in adults if the diagnosis is doubtful, obtain comparison views of the normal side. It is often technically useful to x-ray the clearly labeled normal and abnormal areas side by side on the same film.

Think you see a fracture line, but not sure? Take another view at another angle. Apply stress if indicated. Still in doubt? Immobilize the injured area with a splint or plaster and repeat your examination in a day or two. During that time, your films can be reviewed by an orthopedic consultant.

Treat the patient, not the x-ray. X-rays only tell the structure of the story, omitting vital details of muscle, ligaments, and tendons. The patient with a severely injured painful joint needs immobilization regardless of the negative x-ray findings.

Skull fractures underscore the importance of physical findings over x-ray. A youngster with a linear skull fracture may be alert and happy, while another victim of head trauma whose skull appears normal on x-ray may show vomiting, disorientation, or coma. So, take your x-rays, look at them yourself, but don't forget that these are merely photographs of your patient. Trust your clinical judgment before x-rays. Be a doctor, not a photographer.

The **basilar skull fracture** involving the cribriform plate of the ethmoid may not be visible on x-ray examination, but announces its presence by dripping cerebrospinal fluid from the nose. Does the patient have a fracture or simple rhinorrhea? Here's how to tell. Test the nasal discharge with a urinary dip-stick, such as Hemacombistix. A watery nasal discharge does not contain glucose, but cerebrospinal fluid does. A positive response to the test for glucose in the watery nasal drainage of your head trauma patient is presumptive evidence of a fracture of the cribriform plate of the ethmoid bone.

A **fracture of the orbital floor** may be caused by a baseball, a dashboard, or a clenched fist. Considerable local tenderness and swelling will result, but these will subside spontaneously. Double vision is the key; direct the patient's gaze up, down, right, and left. Does he see a double image in any direction? If so, suspect a blow-out fracture of the orbital floor and order your x-rays accordingly.

Rib fractures are detected by the bent-bow test. Contusions of the rib hurt almost as much as fractures, and local tenderness is an unreliable diagnostic sign. Test for the fractured rib by compressing the sternum and thoracic spine together with the hands, flexing the ribs (Fig. 7–1). The resulting slight rib flexion is painless to bruised ribs, but causes exquisite pain at a fracture site.

Metacarpal fractures can also be detected by indirect pressure. Direct palpation of the injured area will predictably elicit pain, whether or not the metacarpal is fractured. Percuss the distal metacarpal (the knuckle) (Fig. 7–2). This procedure is painless with a contusion, but causes dramatic pain at the site of a metacarpal fracture.

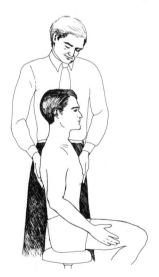

Fig. 7–1. Test for rib fracture by flexing the ribs.

A fracture of the carpal navicular is often missed on x-ray examination, even in the special navicular view. Pain may be minimal, but a missed diagnosis can cause prolonged disability. Look for tenderness of

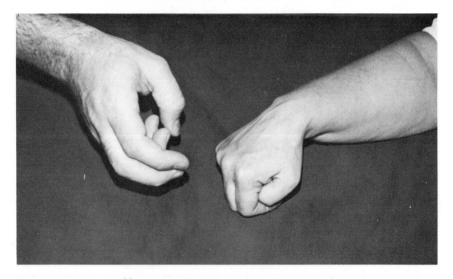

Fig. 7–2. Test for metacarpal fracture by percussing the knuckle.

the anatomic snuffbox. If present, don't trust the first x-rays. The suspected fracture of the carpal navicular should be immobilized and reexamined with x-rays a week later.

The **fractured hip,** the Waterloo of senior citizens, can result from nothing more than a sudden turn of the body. Down goes the patient, lying on the floor, where you find him when summoned to the home. Of course, the hip is tender; he just had a bad fall. But is it bruised or broken? Check the foot. If it is externally rotated, the patient probably has a fractured hip or has suffered a stroke. Further physical examination should exclude evidence of a cerebrovascular accident. Next, internally rotate the foot 60° to normal position. If the hip is bruised, minimal discomfort will result; if it is fractured, the motion will produce severe pain.

ACTIVITIES CAUSING ORTHOPEDIC PROBLEMS

In *Diseases of Workers,* Bernardino Ramazzini (1633–1714) wrote: "When you come to a patient's house, you should ask him what sort of pains he has, what caused them, how many days he has been ill, whether the bowels are working and what sort of food he eats. So says Hippocrates in his work *Affectations.* 'I may venture to add one more question: What occupation does he follow?' " Awkward motions at work and play create orthopedic problems for the physician. When presented with an obscure muscular pain, ask the patient, "What sort of work do you do?" "Have you been doing any heavy lifting?" "Any unusual exercise?" "Can you think of any activity that might have caused your pain?"

Low back strain is the curse of the working man and compensation insurance carriers. Man is structurally engineered to walk on all fours, and his assumption of the upright stature puts an undue strain on the low back musculature. Forward flexion of the spine creates a force arm with a fulcrum at the waist, increasing leverage on the muscles of the low back. Add weight and the leverage often exceeds the strength of low back muscles and ligaments.

Strained muscles protest with painful spasm, causing loss of the normal lumbar lordosis and limiting forward flexion at the base of the spine. A pelvic tilt may be noted and a knot of contracted muscle is often felt along the lumbar spine. The low back strain victim moves carefully, guarding the muscles against further strain.

The treatment of low back strain has changed little since the time of Hippocrates. Electronic devices and pharmaceutical advances are merely refinements of the traditional therapy of all muscle strains: rest, heat, and analgesia. For the back strain victim, rest means being off the feet in bed. Work is prohibited. Bathroom privileges are allowed in less severe cases. Heat may be administered by hot packs, ultrasound, diathermy, heating pad, or old-fashioned hot water bottle. They all work. If the patient uses a heating pad, he should be cautioned not to fall asleep with the pad in place, lest a burn develop. Analgesia for the patient with low back strain varies from aspirin to meperidine (Demerol), perhaps supplemented by a muscle relaxant, such as carisoprodol (Soma).

Cervical sprain, bread and butter of plaintiffs' attorneys, can be caused by lifting a child, turning the head while backing a car into the garage, or twisting the neck during sleep. The basic principles of rest, heat, and analgesia apply. Consider a cervical collar to rest the neck, and if you use ultrasound therapy on the neck, avoid the carotid sinus lest syncope occur.

Rhomboid muscle strain occurs when forced forward extension of the arm pulls the scapula away from the thoracic spine. Has your patient been pushing a car, reaching for a package on a high shelf, or stretching to answer the telephone on a night table too far from the bed? Again prescribe heat, rest, and analgesia, and prohibit lifting and carrying.

A **muscle strain of the groin** results from forced extension of the leg. Is your patient a waitress who repeatedly kicks open a swinging door?

Cervical radiculitis may be due to osteoarthritic spurs or a herniated nucleus pulposus, but a less well known cause is repeated hyperextension of the neck to accommodate to bifocals. (Fig. 7–3). Has your middle-aged patient just been fitted with new bifocal corrective lenses?

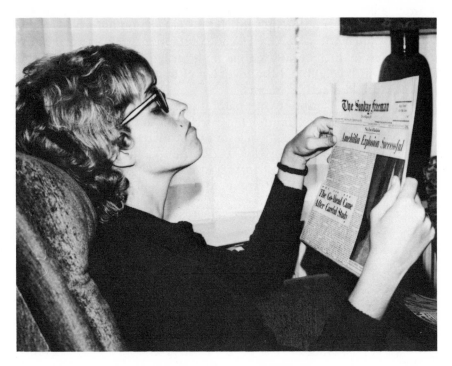

Fig. 7–3. Hyperextension of the neck to accommodate to bifocal lenses can cause cervical radiculitis.

PLASTER AS AN ORTHOPEDIC TOOL

Plaster of Paris is the backbone of orthopedic therapy, allowing solid immobilization of injuries but presenting the potential for equally solid circulatory obstruction. In your casted patients, guard the circulation to the distal extremity and remain ever alert to the danger of arterial occlusion by swelling within an unyielding cast. Caution your patient to call immediately if pallor, numbness, or pain occurs, even if at night or on Sunday afternoon. And when you receive such a call, examine the patient promptly and remove or bivalve the cast if indicated.

Casts do not reduce fractures. Plaster helps maintain the position of fractured fragments, but does not compensate for inadequate reduction. The fracture will heal exactly as you cast it, and if the fragments are improperly aligned at casting, they will be improperly aligned at cast removal 6 weeks later.

Applying the cast is a messy business. Unless you enjoy picking plaster from under your fingernails the rest of the day, don unsterile examination gloves when ready to begin. If you really want to get the bare-hand feel of it, you can use mineral oil to remove the plaster from your hands when finished.

Padding between the stockinet and plaster allows for swelling and facilitates eventual cast removal. Don't skimp, or you may have to replace the cast because of tightness. Proper padding prevents sores caused by plaster grinding on unprotected skin.

Wetting the plaster is an art. The water should be slightly warm; if it is too hot or too cold, the plaster sets poorly. Dip your roll in confidently, holding one end free, allowing all air bubbles to escape. Then wring gently—not too hard or you wring out all the plaster; not too gently or excessive water will delay setting. Don't even try to train a nurse to wet your plaster for you; she'll never do it to suit you.

Drying the cast is hastened by the heat of a nearby gooseneck lamp. Make sure the patient doesn't lean on the wet plaster, solidifying a dent in your fine cast. Don't let the patient out of your sight until his cast is dry.

Getting the patient home after casting may involve some sartorial alterations. Upper extremity casts can be supported with a sling and tucked under the shirt, but knee or ankle casts offer more problems. While the lower extremity cast is drying, the patient or his mother can use your bandage scissors to split trousers carefully up the seam. Once home, buttons with buttonholes or a zipper may be sewn in place, giving the patient at least one pair of trousers that will fit over his cast.

Continued pain after casting is a danger sign. The properly reduced, adequately rested fracture should cause minimal discomfort once casted. Limb elevation and aspirin may be necessary, but severe intractable pain suggests complications. Is the reduction incomplete? Have the fracture fragments shifted during casting? Has swelling within the cast blocked circulation? Is poorly padded plaster rubbing a bony prominence? Is your cast just plain too tight? Examine the patient carefully, take x-rays (several views) through the cast, and don't hesitate to remove the cast if you are in doubt.

Cast removal can be a terrifying experience for a child. The youngster sees the cast cutter as a huge buzz saw about to dismember him.

Tell him what you are going to do. Gain his confidence. Explain that the cast cutter moves back and forth rather than around like a cutting saw; then demonstrate your confidence in the saw's safety by holding the oscillating blade against your forearm. It won't cut you—really. A brief explanation and demonstration help gain the child's cooperation.

MAJOR JOINT INJURIES

The **dislocated shoulder** may be encountered at home, the patient lying on the floor having crawled painfully to the telephone to call his doctor. Confirm the presence of a glenohumeral dislocation by palpating the head of the humerus anteriorly, noting absence of the greater tuberosity below the acromion, and demonstrating the patient's inability to place the hand of the involved side on the opposite shoulder. Shoulder dislocations are best reduced early before muscle spasm occurs. Leave the patient on the floor, remove your shoe, and apply countertraction with your foot in the patient's axilla. Wrap a towel around the patient's arm to absorb perspiration, and pull firmly. Don't expend all your strength in an initial burst of enthusiasm; about 5 minutes of sustained traction will be needed. Gradually, muscle spasm is overcome and the dislocation is reduced with a reassuring pop as the humeral head returns to the glenoid cavity. Bring the arm to the side and apply a Velpeau dressing; then check your results with x-ray. The Velpeau dressing should be worn for 3 weeks. After that, shoulder motion should gradually be increased to normal.

A **fracture of the neck of the humerus** usually requires no manipulation, but prolonged immobilization can result in a frozen shoulder, in spite of flawless fracture healing. A sling and swathe prevent motion at the fracture site, allowing shoulder exercises to begin as soon as acute pain has subsided. By the end of 3 weeks, the sling and swathe can usually be discarded.

Shoulder exercises prevent and treat the frozen shoulder. As with all joint exercises, a full range of motion is imperative, including passive and hopefully active movements. Beware the patient who seems to have 90 degree abduction at the shoulder, but is really moving only his scapula and spine.

DonTigny (1970) described four exercises for stretching the shoulder into lateral rotation, flexion, abduction-elevation, and extension, moving the body in relation to the arm, which is stabilized on a table (Figs. 7–4 through 7–7). Lateral rotation is achieved with the patient sitting parallel to the table, flexing the elbow, resting the forearm on the edge

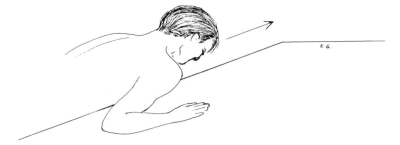

Fig. 7–4. Shoulder exercises: lateral rotation.

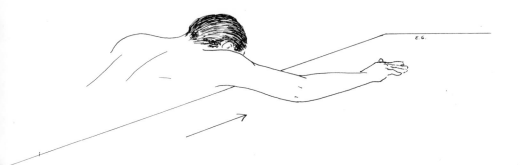

Fig. 7–5. Shoulder exercises: flexion.

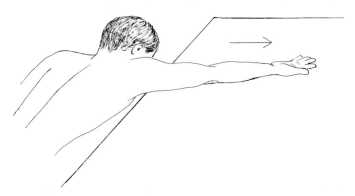

Fig. 7–6. Shoulder exercises: abduction-elevation.

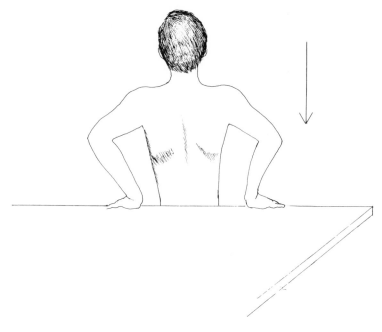

Fig. 7–7. Shoulder exercises: extension.

of the table, and leaning forward from the waist, bringing the head down to the table level. The same position is used for flexion, resting the forearm along the table, moving the arm forward while bending from the waist. Abduction-elevation is accomplished with the patient seated parallel to the table and the forearm resting, palm up, toward the other side of the table; the patient flexes the trunk laterally, sliding the arm across the table, bringing the head down to the arm. Extension is accomplished with the patient standing, back to the table, grasping the edge of the table with both hands and squatting slightly with flexed elbows, extending the shoulders.

If necessary, tight shoulder muscles may be loosened by preceding the exercises with Hydrocollator, ultrasound, or diathermy treatment. A muscle relaxant, such as orphenadrine (Norflex), 100 mg, may also help loosen tight shoulder musculature.

The **supracondylar fracture** of the humerus is an evil injury. The deformity is usually obvious upon observation of the elbow (Fig. 7–8); don't try to make the diagnosis by manipulation. Check for arterial or nerve damage (in case someone asks you later), support the injured elbow gently on a pillow, and bundle the patient off to your best orthopedic consultant.

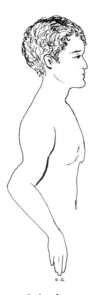

Fig. 7–8. Supracondylar fracture of the humerus.

The **sprained wrist** is as common as chronic appendicitis. Be skeptical. Take careful x-rays, including oblique and navicular views. If the x-rays are unrevealing but the injury apparently severe, immobilize the wrist in plaster or at least an Ace bandage, support it with a sling, and reexamine with x-rays 4 or 5 days later.

The **sprained ankle** can cause the patient as much trouble as a fracture. Your x-rays should include a stressed view of the ankle. There are many ways to treat the sprained ankle, including plaster, the soft cast, tape, or an elastic bandage, but all include the important principle of not bearing weight. This means crutches. Immobilize the ankle with your favorite method and see that the patient is carefully fitted with crutches and instructed in their proper use. Don't let him spend 3 weeks walking on his axillae. Reexamine the sprained ankle at weekly intervals and allow gradual resumption of weight-bearing once the ankle is pain-free. The high-school athlete should remain on the bench for 1 month after the severe sprained ankle seems well.

Knee injuries abound in football, skiing, and other active sports. Many a young athlete has sacrificed a meniscus for the greater glory of his local high school. Be conservative in your prognosis of the knee injury; if two patients come to your office the same day, one with a fractured lateral malleolus and the other with a twisted knee, your fractured ankle patient will be schussing the slopes in a few months while the knee injury patient is still limping around the ski lodge.

Knee injuries may involve a torn meniscus, a strained medial collateral ligament, or both. Swelling and pain cloud the initial evaluation, and x-rays are rarely revealing. Most severe twisting knee injuries are best immobilized with a cylinder cast or at least a posterior splint supplemented by crutches. Maintain immobilization for 3 to 6 weeks in the best of cases, and prohibit sports for about 3 months.

The well-publicized instant surgery on knee injuries of professional athletes is justified by economic considerations. The star quarterback can't afford to be out of action while his knee injury slowly heals. The high-school athlete can; don't be in a rush to open his knee. Give conservative therapy a fair trial.

Aspiration of the knee joint is a technically simple procedure. The key to success is seating the patient on the examination table, allowing the weight of the leg to open the knee joint (Fig. 7–9). After careful scrubbing, anesthetize the skin with 1 ml of 1% lidocaine (Xylocaine) and insert an 18-gauge needle into the joint just below the patella. Aspirate the synovial fluid or blood, inject steroids if indicated, and cover the injection site with a small Band-Aid.

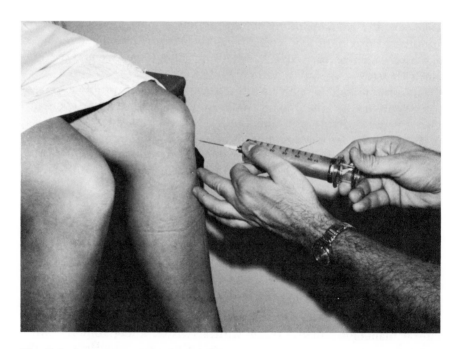

Fig. 7–9. Aspiration of the knee joint.

INJURIES TO FINGERS AND TOES

Digital joint dislocations are common in active children with loose ligaments. Reduction is easily attained by firm traction on the digit distal to the dislocation (Fig. 7–10). Once reduced, the joint should be splinted for 3 weeks to allow healing of damaged ligaments.

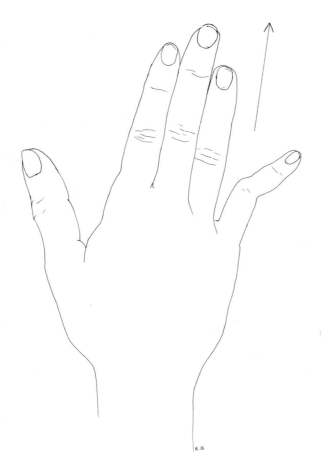

Fig. 7–10. Reduction of digital joint dislocation.

Chip fractures of the fingers are caused by baseballs, volleyballs, and basketballs. Attempted manipulation of the chip is unwarranted. Splint the digit for 3 weeks. After that prescribe graded exercise to gradually restore normal movement at the joint. There can be no justification for referring these simple chip fractures to an already overburdened orthopedic surgeon.

Digital fractures in toddlers rarely require more than splinting. If the two fragments are in the same room, they will get together and heal. But your standard aluminum splints are all adult size; splint the tiny finger with a paperclip, either regular size or giant size, secured with adhesive tape. Three weeks of immobilization is plenty.

Fractured toes heal well no matter what you do. The great toe can be splinted with a short aluminum finger-type splint, usually discarded after 10 to 14 days. A fractured smaller toe is padded and taped to its neighbor. Hard-soled footwear is recommended; usually the top of the shoe must be cut to prevent pressure on the fracture.

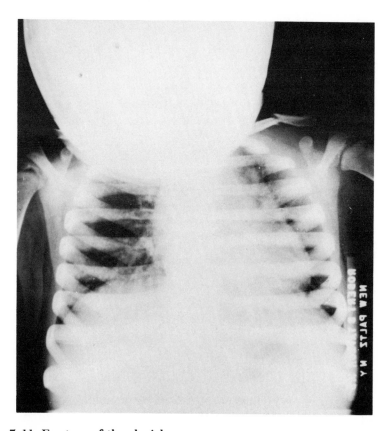

Fig. 7–11. Fracture of the clavicle.

ORTHOPEDIC INJURIES OF CHILDREN

The **fractured clavicle** occurs when Johnny falls from a tree or out of bed. Johnny won't move his arm. The fracture site is tender to palpa-

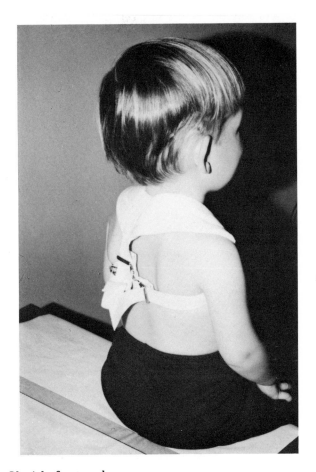

Fig. 7–12. Clavicle fracture brace.

tion. Direct the x-ray beam from slightly cephalad to the prone patient. In a squirming infant, you may not get more than one film, so use a large plate and include both sides. The fracture is usually obvious upon examination of the x-ray film (Fig. 7–11).

The treatment of clavicular fractures is simple, and orthopedic referral should not be needed. Caution the parents that, no matter how treated, a permanent lump of callus will develop at the fracture site. Explain how holding the shoulders back pulls the fracture fragments into alignment; then apply a Meek's clavicle brace (Fig. 7–12) and leave it in place for 3 weeks. Within 3 or 4 days, the youngster no longer complains of pain. Check your patient weekly, adjusting the clavicle brace as necessary. At the end of 3 weeks, the Meek's brace is discarded, and if Johnny will stay out of the apple tree for 2 months more, final healing will occur uneventfully.

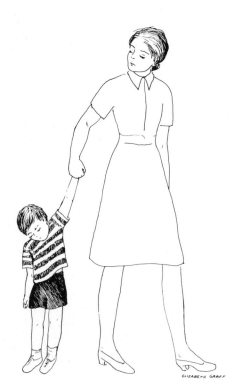

Fig. 7–13. The sudden tug that causes nursemaid's elbow.

"**Nursemaid's elbow**", a subluxation of the radial head, occurs when mother jerks her child back sharply by his outstretched arm (Fig. 7–13), causing the cartilaginous radial head to partially slide out of its encircling ligament. The youngster guards the arm, and attempted pronation and supination at the wrist are met with loud complaints. X-ray examination shows no fracture, but also usually fails to reveal the subluxation because the radial head is not ossified in youngsters.

The subluxated radial head is easily reduced in the office without anesthesia. Seat the child in the mother's lap and tell her to hold him tight. Gradually, turn the elbow into full supination, followed by deliberate flexion of the elbow. As the elbow is flexed, the radial head pops back into place with an audible snap. The reduction is quite stable, and unless there has been associated severe trauma, immobilization is unnecessary.

Painful knees, usually dismissed as growing pains, may be due to flat feet—pronation of the foot with eversion of the heel. The foot deformity causes an abnormal stress on the ankle and knee. Flat feet, of course, are a hereditary uncorrectable deformity, but the resulting symptoms can be relieved by proper footwear. Prescribe good quality, hard-soled, Oxford shoes with scaphoid pads to support the arch and 3/16-inch heel wedges to prevent eversion of the heel.

Muscular dystrophy is one of those rare diseases that you may encounter seldom, if ever. Like other rare diseases, the incidence may be one in a million, but to the victim, the incidence is 100 percent. Tuck this diagnostic tip into the back files of your memory: The child who can't squat and stand again without using his arms may have muscular dystrophy.

References and Suggestions for Further Reading

1. Berne C J, Rosoff L: Symposium on trauma. Surg Clin North Am 48:1185–1477, 1968.
2. Cailliet R: Hand Pain and Impairment. Philadelphia, Davis, 1971.
3. Chamberlain G V: Backache. Br Med J 2:99–100, 1971.
4. Cozen L N: Orthopedic examination of the infant and child. Am Fam Physician GP 4:60–65, 1971.
5. Crenshaw A H: Campbell's Operative Orthopedics. St Louis, Mosby, 1963.
6. DonTigny R L: Passive shoulder exercises. Phys Ther 50:1707–1709, 1970.
7. Ferguson A B Jr: Orthopedic Surgery in Infancy and Childhood. Baltimore, Williams & Wilkins, 1968.
8. Kraus H: Clinical Treatment of Back and Neck Pain. New York, McGraw-Hill, 1970.
9. Nicholas J A: Injuries to knee ligaments. JAMA 212:2236–2239, 1970.

10. Shires G T: Care of the Trauma Patient. New York, McGraw-Hill, 1966.

11. Turek S L : Orthopaedics: Principles and Their Applications, 3rd ed. Philadelphia, Lippincott, 1967.

12. Zuidema G: Trauma. Philadelphia, Saunders, 1967.

8

Uncomplicated Urology

As men draw near the common goal
Can anything be sadder
Than he who, master of his soul,
Is servant to his bladder?

The Speculum
Melbourne, No. 140 (1938)

Filtration of the blood with removal of waste products in a liquid vehicle sounds like an elementary exercise in hydrodynamics, and when functioning properly, the urinary tract efficiently controls the body's fluid and chemical balance. Unfortunately, abnormalities of the urinary tract are so common that one wonders if the system has yet been perfected.

PEDIATRIC UROLOGY

Enuresis is why Billy can't go to camp and Mary can't sleep over at her friend's home. All infants have enuresis, but sometime between ages 2 and 5 years, most youngsters achieve volitional bladder control. Some have better control than others, and half of all normal 4-year-old children have enuresis at some time. Unless complicated by frequency, dysuria, pyuria, or other evidence of infection, you need not worry about the child with enuresis until he passes 5 years of age.

Enuresis is usually emotional in origin, reflecting resentment of a younger sibling, fantasies of rejection, or a desire for infantile dependence. However, enuresis is occasionally caused by a surgically correctable urinary tract abnormality which, if neglected during childhood, could lead to irreparable renal damage. Be suspicious of the youngster with urinary tract infections, a history of urologic abnormalities in the family, daytime urinary incontinence, and failure to respond to therapy. Examine a freshly passed urine specimen at each visit. Watch the boy with enuresis pass urine; a splayed or narrow stream may point to a urethral abnormality. If you suspect overt urinary tract pathology, refer the child for urologic evaluation including voiding cystourethrography.

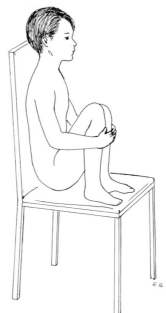

Fig. 8–1. Knee-chest position that forces testes to descend into scrotum.

Emotionally triggered enuresis has been treated with imipramine (Tofranil), ephedrine, and propantheline (Pro-Banthine), with varying degrees of success. Here's a tip: Help the child increase his bladder capacity by drinking large quantities of water and holding his urine as long as possible. Upon finally voiding, he should measure the output and write it down, keeping score as the bladder volume increases.

A **varicocele** is usually encountered upon routine physical examination of young boys. I can't recall a varicocele as a presenting complaint. If the condition is mentioned at all, reassure the patient and his family that the varicocele is a normal variant—simple varicose veins of the scrotum. But remember that the "normal" varicocele is on the left; a right-sided varicocele may indicate pelvic pressure causing increased venous stasis in the scrotum and deserves further evaluation.

The **undescended testicle,** like the varicocele, is usually detected upon routine examination. Many apparently undescended testicles are temporarily hiding in the inguinal canal; the most common cause of an empty scrotum is the doctor's cold hand. Here's a good confirming test: Seat the young lad in a straight-backed chair and instruct him to hug his knees to his chest (Fig. 8–1). This posture causes pressure on the inguinal canal, forcing the testes into the scrotum.

The undescended testicle can be treated expectantly with safety until age 5. Occasionally, a course of chorionic gonadotropin injections is warranted but rarely successful. Before puberty, the inguinal canal should be surgically explored and the testes brought down into the scrotum.

UROLOGIC TRAUMA

Zipper injuries of the penis are painful. Your patient is usually a child, rushed in by his frantic mother, the loose penile skin entwined in a closed zipper. Resist the temptation to inject the area full of lidocaine, causing edema. Instead, sedate the youngster with your favorite tranquilizer and rub in liberal quantities of Nupercainal ointment. Cut the entire zipper free from the trousers, allowing unhampered manipulation. Then, with the patient sedated and the skin at least partially anesthetized with Nupercainal ointment, close slightly, then open the zipper. Do it fast! It hurts. Learn from the experience of others: Don't try to pry open the zipper closure; it is well made and won't budge. Also, don't cut across the zipper, preventing its subsequent opening.

Urethral injuries result from falling astride a fence or bicycle bar. Severe pain confounds evaluation, but does not negate the physician's responsibility to detect urethral injury before urine passage. Failure to diagnose the torn urethra floods the tissues with necrosing urine, causing extensive local damage. Here is one instance where a urologic diagnosis must be made without benefit of urine analysis. If suspicious, catheterize the patient with an indwelling Foley catheter, to be left in place until you are sure no urethral defect remains.

CATHETERS AND THEIR PROBLEMS

Catheters, dilators, and sounds are valuable instruments in the hands of a skilled urologist, but fiendish torture devices when wielded by an inexperienced intern. Whenever you insert a catheter or sound, remember there's a patient attached to the other end.

Unless you have considerable experience in urologic instrumentation, send the patient with a tight stricture to a consultant.

Prostatic obstruction can thwart attempted catheterization. A metal obturator, even if you have one in the office, presents the danger of a false passage. There's an easier way to overcome an obstructing prostate: Use the bulb of the Foley catheter as a dilator, partially filling the 5-ml bag when obstruction is encountered (Fig. 8–2). Be sure to use plenty of lidocaine jelly. The bulb hydrodilator can prevent considerable urethral trauma.

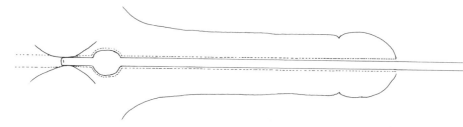

Fig. 8–2. A Foley catheter with partially filled bulb dilates urethra obstructed by enlarged prostate.

The **Foley catheter bulb that won't deflate** is usually blocked by sediment acting as a ball-valve. Try to burst the bag by injecting several syringefuls of sterile water. If this maneuver is unsuccessful, the injection of 5 ml of ordinary ether through the tubing into the bulb is usually followed promptly by bulb deflation and easy catheter removal.

Maintaining a catheter at home is a formidable undertaking for any family—almost impossible unless one household member has had special training. Truly, indwelling catheter maintenance should be managed in a nursing home, although as we will see in Chapter 10, Medicare doesn't agree. If at all possible, correct the patient's need for indwelling catheterization by medical or surgical means. Take a chance on your 79-year-old patient's ability to withstand prostatectomy; he will probably do just fine. Nevertheless, some senior citizens require permanent catheterization and cannot afford nursing home care; the only alternative is home care of the catheter.

The same principles of sterility apply at home as in the hospital. Use aseptic technique when inserting the catheter. Instruct the family in irrigation with sterile water or saline, and stress the importance of boiling the Asepto syringe after use. Prescribe a urinary antiseptic, such as methenamine hippurate (Hiprex), a single 1-gm tablet every 12 hours, to prevent infection. If the patient is ambulatory, the catheter may be attached to a Bardex bag strapped to his leg; if he is bedfast, an ordinary 1-gal cider jug on the floor makes a fine receptacle for the urine drained by the catheter.

Bladder training should precede attempted catheter removal. The catheter should be clamped for progressively longer intervals, and the clamp released when the patient reports an urge to void. To determine bladder capacity, measure the urine voided when the clamp is released. When the patient can reliably detect 250–300 ml of urine in the bladder, sensing an urge to void, he is ready for a trial of catheter removal. The patient who fails to verbalize the voiding urge no matter how full the bladder is a poor candidate for catheter removal.

URINARY TRACT INFECTION

Falstaff: . . . What says the doctor to my water?
Page: He said, sir, the water itself was a good healthy water; but, for the party that owed it, he might have moe diseases than he knew for."

William Shakespeare (1564–1616)
HENRY IV, Part II

The urinary tract infection causes an overwhelming urge to void, unrelieved by the passage of a few drops of scalding urine. Up and down all night voiding, suffering with backache and fever, the patient with a urinary tract infection is miserable indeed. The urine contains pus cells and sometimes a little blood. Expensive colony counts are not needed; you know the patient has an infection. The equally expensive urine culture and antibiotic sensitivity testing are also unnecessary in the otherwise uncomplicated first-episode urinary tract infection; by the time your culture report is submitted by the lab, your patient will have been asymptomatic for 3 or 4 days.

The vast majority of urinary tract infections respond promptly to sulfonamides or tetracycline. Save the more costly nitrofurantoin (Furadantin), nalidixic acid (NegGram), and cephaloglycin (Kafocin) for stubborn, resistant infections. The patient with severe dysuria will be grateful for a prescription for phenazopyridine (Pyridium), an azo dye with the twin distinctions of providing urinary tract analgesia and coloring the urine a brilliant orange—the latter may be a source of no little consternation to the patient unless he is forewarned by the doctor.

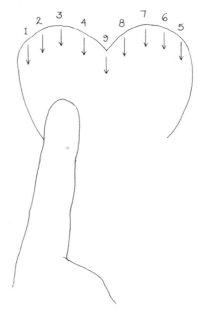

Fig. 8–3. Technique of prostatic massage.

Treat a urinary infection long enough to eradicate it. Pay special attention to the patient with recurrent cystitis. Although certainly an oversimplification, it has been recommended that the first urinary tract infection be treated for 2 weeks, the second for 2 months and the third for 2 years. One 1-gm Hiprex tablet morning and night may spare the cystitis patient the torment of recurrent urinary tract infections.

PROSTATITIS

Prostatitis is a disease of traveling salesmen, bus drivers, and other men who spend long hours behind the wheel of a motor vehicle: The prolonged sitting plus the vibration of the machine result in congestion of the prostate. If infection occurs, failure of the prostate to drain efficiently leads to chronic disease with recurrence and persistence of symptoms. Treat infectious prostatitis patients with your antibiotic of choice. Many patients respond to 150 mg of demeclocycline (Declomycin) or 1 gm of sulfisoxazole (Gantrisin) four times daily for 10 days.

The prostatitis victim should avoid long motor trips and alcoholic beverages, both capable of producing acute, painful flare-ups. Regular sexual relations help empty the prostate gland of secretions, but sexual excitation without ejaculation should be avoided. As with any infection, heat is beneficial, usually prescribed as a prolonged hot tub bath.

Prostatic massage helps remove sluggish prostatic secretions and is usually performed at weekly intervals while the patient is symptomatic. Learn the proper technique for prostatic massage: use slow strokes from above down, proceeding from laterally to medially over each lobe and ending with firm midline strokes forcing prostatic secretions down the urethra (Fig. 8–3).

Prostatic fluid, expressed by massage, should be examined microscopically on a clean slide. No staining is necessary. Under low power, check the number of white blood cells. Normal prostatic fluid contains 20 to 40 white blood cells per low-power field; more than 40 indicates infection of the prostate gland.

UROLOGIC EMERGENCIES

Paraphimosis, as the patient will tell you, is a urologic emergency of the first order. Often the constriction can be reduced by the local application of ice, followed by manual compression of the glands for 5 to 10 minutes, along with gentle traction on the prepuce. If this is unsuccessful, inject 150 TRU (turbidity reducing units) of hyaluronidase around the constricting ring, apply ice, and try again. Still unsuccessful? Then you should refer the patient to your urologic consultant for reduction under general anesthesia.

Torsion of the testicle causes arterial occlusion and requires prompt surgery if the testicle is to be saved. Fortunately, severe pain prompts immediate medical consultation. Rise to the emergency. Don't apply ice, prescribe antibiotics, or try any other time-wasting maneuvers. Rush the patient to a waiting consultant and the operating room.

Kidney stones nestle peacefully in the renal pelvis, causing symptoms only when one migrates to the bladder. Sudden flank pain accompanied by microscopic hematuria announces the stone's departure. Every inch of the journey is marked by colicky pain radiating to the groin. There may be point tenderness over the stone's locus in the ureter.

Administer meperidine (Demerol), encourage the patient to drink fluids, and let him walk around; Motion and gravity enhance the stone's progression. Most ureteral stones are tiny and their exit will be overlooked unless the urine is strained. The nylon stretch material in white panty hose has a fine mesh, is easily stretched over a urinal or bedpan, and is ideal for stone-catching.

Most ureteral stones will be passed within a few days, but laggards will require instrumentation or surgery.

Stone analysis is an oft-neglected diagnostic test with important implications. Most kidney stones can be related to chronic pyelonephritis, calcium, cystine, or uric acid. Of course, chronic renal infection should be treated with antibiotics and forced consumption of 3 liters of fluid daily. Calcium stones should prompt reduction of intake of calcium-containing dairy products and a search for possible hyperparathyroidism.

Recurrence of cystine calculus may be prevented by alkalinization of the urine. The patient should take sodium bicarbonate, three 660-mg tablets three or four times daily and test his urine frequently with nitrazine paper, maintaining a urinary pH of 7.0 or above. This patient too should drink 3 liters of fluids daily.

Uric acid calculi can also be prevented by alkalinizing the urine with sodium bicarbonate tablets and monitoring urinary pH with nitrazine paper. In addition, the patient should be tested for gout and should eliminate from his diet purine-rich foods, including sweetbreads, liver, sardines, anchovies, and kidneys. Hyperuricemia is treated with allopurinol (Zyloprim), 100 mg one to three times daily, with dose adjustment to maintain a normal blood uric acid level.

References and Suggestions for Further Reading

1.   Albers D D, Stalcup O L Jr: Carcinoma of the prostate in private practice. J Okla State Med Assoc 64:57–59, 1971.

2.   Allan W R, Brown R B: Torsion of the testis: A review of 58 cases. Br Med J 1:-1396–1397, 1966.

3.   Harrison J H, Perlmutter A D: Major urological emergencies. Surg Clin North Am 46:685–712, 1966.

4.   Holland M E, Hurwitz L M, Nice C M Jr: Traumatic lesions of the urinary tract. Radiol Clin North Am 4:433–450, 1966.

5.   Mostofi F K, Smith D E: The Kidney. Baltimore, Williams & Wilkins, 1966.

6.   Murphy S, Nickols J, Umphress A, Hammar S, Eddy R, Chapman W: Adolescent enuresis: A multiple contingency hypothesis. JAMA 218:1189–1191 1971.

7.   Norden C W, Kass E H: Bacteriuria of pregnancy: A critical appraisal. Annu Rev Med 19:431–470, 1968.

8.   Pitts R F: Physiology of the Kidney and Body Fluids. Chicago, Year Book, 1968.

9. Rangno R E, McLeod P J, Ruedy J, Ogilvie R I: Treatment of benign prostatic hypertrophy with medrogestone. Clin Pharmacol Ther 12:658–665, 1971.

10. Symposium on renal disorders. Pediatr Clin North Am 11:515–766, 1964.

11. Symposium on the problems of prostatic obstruction. Br J Surg 52:744–760, 1965.

12. Vaughan E D Jr, Alfert H J, Gillenwater J Y: Obstructive uropathy secondary to phimosis and balanoposthitis. Am J Dis Child 120:72–73, 1970.

13. Wesson L G: Physiology of the Human Kidney. New York, Grune & Stratton, 1969.

9

Gentle Gynecology

The surgical cycle in woman: Appendix removed, right kidney hooked up, gallbladder taken out, gastro-enterostomy, clean sweep of uterus and adnexa.

Aphorisms
Sir William Osler (1849–1919)

Women love their husbands, adore their sons, but worship their gynecologists. The true joy of gynecology, as any other medical specialty, springs from the day by day 60-hour week of relieving patient suffering—palliating pruritic vulvae, arbitrating marital woes, and planning procreation at a convenient time.

THE PELVIC EXAMINATION

The pelvic examination, oft-repeated, wears deep ruts of habit. Make sure your habits are good ones.

An anxious patient, anticipating the pelvic examination, may show tachycardia, elevated blood pressure, and tremor of the hands. If your patient seems unduly nervous, perform the internal examination first, then proceed with the general examination, the patient relieved that the worst part is out of the way.

Illumination of the vagina and cervix presents several options. An electric head lamp allows direct illumination, can be focused, and is a superior method if the cord does not become tangled in the stirrups of the examining table. Use of an incandescent bulb and head mirror requires practice, but can provide excellent illumination. Tucked under the examiner's chin, the traditional gooseneck lamp also provides adequate illumination.

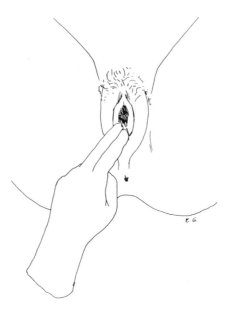

Fig. 9–1. Depress the posterior fornix before introducing the speculum into the vagina.

Warm the vaginal speculum by holding the blades in your hand while the nurse drapes the patient. Even better, keep your metal specula on a heating pad or in an incubator box—an old cigar humidor equipped with a night-light bulb works admirably. Although ecologically indefensible, plastic vaginal specula have the advantages of no clean-up, no autoclaving, and no coldness.

The **external genitalia** should be observed before you insert the speculum. Gently spread the labia; observe the urethral meatus. Ask the patient to "bear down as though you were having a bowel movement" and, cautious while the patient performs this maneuver, check the vaginal support.

Introduce the speculum gently. First depress the posterior fornix with two fingers (Fig. 9–1) telling the patient to "let this muscle relax." If it's still tight, tell her to squeeze your two fingers tight until the muscles fatigue; then she *has to* relax. In an older woman, bearing down exposes the lower anterior and posterior vaginal walls; lay the speculum between them and relaxation will pull it past the introitus. In a younger woman, the vagina must be entered with the speculum blades placed diagonally, avoiding painful pressure on the labia.

The **cervix** is exposed and material obtained for the Papaucolaou test by gently scraping the endocervix with a spatula or a cotton-tipped applicator and transferring the scrapings to a slide. The cotton-tipped applicator is much less likely to provoke the bleeding that negates the test. If the cervix is irritated and dry, a drop of glycerine on the spatula or applicator may prevent bleeding.

The **fundus and adnexa** are gently palpated using bimanual examination. Think about the layers of tissue (and possibly fat) you are feeling through; the ovary that can be accurately outlined is probably enlarged. Avoid squeezing the ovary; it hurts.

The **rectal examination** is as important as the vaginal, outlining uterine fibroids, adnexal masses, and rectal growths. Before inserting your probing digit, warn the patient, "Now I am going to examine your rectum. This will hurt a little," because it does.

THERAPY IN GYNECOLOGY

Recurrent vaginitis plagues many women and gynecologists. Of course, you will consider the usual causes—monilial, trichomonal, and bacterial infections. Here are some other factors to consider. Oral contraceptives predispose to vaginitis, particularly moniliasis. The husband may be reinfecting his wife each time you think her vaginitis is cured. Treat him too. Tampons may cause an inflammatory reaction and are a common source of vaginitis. The pinworm is sometimes the culprit. Sensitizing vaginal jellies, including mercuric compounds and those containing paraben preservatives, may be responsible for vaginitis.

Painful sexual relations are not fun. Once vaginal infections have been excluded, a common cause of dyspareunia is faulty sexual technique. Give the patient (and/or her husband) the benefit of your knowledge and experience. Explain the importance of foreplay, clitoral stimulation, and mutual responsiveness. The sex act is neither a duel nor a race. Slow, measured concern for the partner's pleasure, supplemented by a clinical understanding of proper technique, will usually overcome dyspareunia.

Fertility is a cooperative venture, and although it is usually the wife who brings the problem of sterility to her physician, the husband is subfertile at least half the time. Failure to conceive is usually a result of deficiencies in both partners; this is documented by the prompt overt evidence of fertility when a "sterile" man or woman remarries. Avoid fixing blame on one partner.

The subfertile male may respond to the empiric prescription of thyroid hormone, 1 or 2 gr daily. Some may prove fertile following treatment with chorionic gonadotropin (APL), 5000 units injected intramuscularly three times weekly for 6 to 8 weeks. Limiting sexual relations to once weekly may allow an increased build-up of sperm.

The subfertile female may unwittingly prevent conception by using spermicidal douches or vaginal jelly, or by arising from bed immediately following intercourse so that the ejaculate falls from the cervix. A flat basal body temperature "curve" indicates anovulatory cycles. In most cases, the evaluation of the subfertile female falls outside the province of the family physician and should be referred to a specialist in the field.

Venereal warts are often treated with 25% podophyllin in tincture of benzoin, removed by copious flushing after 5 hours. Impress your patient with this fact: The podophyllin must be removed. If it is applied vaginally, have the patient return and flush the vaginal wall yourself if you doubt her dexterity with a douche bag. Left undistrubed, podophyllin cauterizes the epithelium after finishing off the wart, resulting in exquisitely painful ulcerations.

The **vaginal douche** has a colorful history in folklore. Postcoital douching, a popular contraception technique before the pill, accounted for many large families in the past. The normal faint odor of pubic apocrine glands has prompted douching, as often as daily, in generations of fastidious women. A variety of techniques have been used, including connecting the tubing directly to the spigot.

Douching is unnecessary for the normal healthy vagina. If the patient insists, she may douche monthly following the menstrual flow and, of course, when prescribed by the doctor for the treatment of vaginitis. The pharmaceutical industry has yet to surpass the efficacy of the traditional vinegar douche—1 oz of white vinegar to each quart of water used.

The proper technique of vaginal douching is as follows: The patient lies on her back in the bathtub, assuming the traditional position for sexual relations. With the douche bag suspended well above the body to provide hydrostatic pressure, the tube is inserted high in the vagina and the clamp released, allowing the fluid to flow freely. Subsequently, the tube is clamped and the vagina allowed to drain. The process is repeated until 1 to 2 qt of fluid have been used.

YOUR YOUNGER FEMALE PATIENTS

Vaginitis in a child suggests a foreign body—peanut, toy, or bead. With the patient's cooperation, the preadolescent vagina can be examined with a nasal speculum lubricated with lidocaine ointment (Fig. 9–2). No foreign body found? Then culture material from the vagina: Include a culture on Nickerson's medium for monilia and a hanging-drop suspension for trichomonas. Most nonspecific pediatric vaginitis responds to nitrofurazone (Furacin) urethral inserts (with or without hydrocortisone) inserted vaginally twice daily.

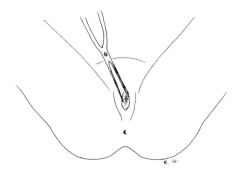

Fig. 9–2. Use a nasal speculum for the pediatric vaginal examination.

The **menstrual flow** of teenagers confounds mothers and grandmothers, who require repeated reassurance by the physician. The 14-year-old girl who has normal budding breasts and incipient axillary hair will begin to menstruate soon; wait a few months. The 15-year-old girl who menstruates once every 3 months is also normal; she is having anovulatory irregular cycles that will stabilize later. The 16-year-old with irregular menstrual periods ranging from 15- to 50-day intervals needs your assurance that her irregular menstrual cycle is not abnormal. The 17-year-old whose periods have been fairly regular for a year or two and who has missed the last two periods probably has another "normal" problem—a normal pregnancy.

Breast development fascinates and worries your pubertal patients, who often wear bras for no other reason than warmth. In general, breast development will follow a family pattern, earlier and more striking in endomorphic girls, later and less luxuriant in ectomorphs. To paraphrase George Orwell, all girls are created equal, but some are more equal than others. To answer the patient's question, there is no safe effective way to increase breast size, and consideration of hormone or silicone treatment should be discouraged. A slight increase in underlying muscle mass will be realized by pectoralis muscle exercises, lying supine on the floor, a book about as heavy as this one held extended to each side, then raised to meet in the midline above the chest.

CONTRACEPTION

Oral contraception is the most reliable method of fertility control available today; it has an excellent safety record, considering the millions of woman-years of clinical experience available. Certainly, oral contraception is the method of choice for nulliparous patients, and many women have used it continuously for 10 to 12 years without untoward effect. Critics of oral contraceptives fail to consider the morbidity and mortality associated with the unwanted pregnancy.

Intrauterine devices have proved their value in America. Coils and shields are best tolerated by multiparous patients. With increasing experience and improved devices, the rejection rate and failure ratio continue to fall.

Diaphragm and jelly, the best contraception method available until 10 years ago, should be recommended only for the woman who has a clinical familiarity with her own internal anatomy. The diaphragm is not for the young bride; by the time she learns to position the diaphragm correctly, she is already pregnant.

The **condom** reliably prevents conception when used by a conscientious, adept male partner. There are few of these. Contraception is not the concern of the average male, and the most reliable contraception methods continue to be those controlled by the female.

Vaginal creams and foams are, at best, a fair means of contraception, recommended only for those couples who would not mind another member of the family.

The **rhythm method** is highly unreliable and recommended only for patients who plan to have a large family.

Teenagers and birth control pills give doctors gray hair. That cute little 15-year-old high-school sophomore tells you she is having regular sexual relations with her 16-year-old pimply-faced boyfriend, and please would you prescribe oral contraceptives. Refuse her on the grounds that she is underage, and you may have to deal with an unwanted pregnancy in a few months. Give her the prescription, and about a week later her mother will storm into the office demanding to know why you have corrupted her daughter. My rule is this: If she is 18 or over and already having sexual relations, I arbitrarily declare her an adult and prescribe the pills. If she is 17 or less, I insist upon parental consent before prescribing oral contraceptives unless marriage is imminent. Maybe my solution is a cop-out, but it keeps the doctor out of trouble.

Clinics, with their impersonal attitudes and lack of doctor-patient relation, are perhaps better equipped to handle contraception requests from underage teenagers. The clinic is not as vulnerable as you are to blame-seeking angry parents of wayward daughters.

PREGNANCY

Pregnancy is the most common cause of amenorrhea and the underlying etiology of many complaints during the childbearing years. The young woman's medical history is incomplete without the question, "When was your last menstrual period?"—a more subtle inquiry than, "Are you pregnant?" If it has indeed been 6 weeks since the last menstrual period, ask "Is there any reason why your period might be late?"

The **pregnancy test** is a useful office procedure. The Pregnosticon slide test is rapid, simple, and highly accurate. What about the equivocal pregnancy test? It may be inconclusive because testing was attempted too early in gestation, but if it was done more than 3 weeks since the missed menstrual period, the equivocal pregnancy test may be the first hint of spontaneous abortion.

Can the sex of the infant be selected? Doctor Landrum B. Shettles, of the Columbia-Presbyterian Medical Center, suggests the following technique, based upon the finding of two types of sperm—small, motile alkaline-active Y-chromosome-bearing androsperm and larger, less motile acidophilic X-chromosome-bearing gynosperm:

For a female infant:
   No intercourse 2 or 3 days prior to ovulation
   Precede intercourse with an acidic vinegar douche
   Avoid female orgasm
   Shallow penetration at the time of orgasm
   Normal or increased sexual frequency until 3 days before ovulation.

For a male infant
   Sexual relations should coincide with ovulation
   Precede intercourse with an alkaline baking soda douche

Attempt to achieve female orgasm

Deep penetration by the male at the time of orgasm

Increase the sperm count by sexual abstinence from the last menstrual period until the day of ovulation

Statistical analysis of Shettles' data reveals an excellent success rate. Suggest this technique to your patients: You'll be right at least 50 percent of the time.

Birth is the most dangerous moment of life. Babies come when least expected. Consider the number of babies born in taxicabs or police cars. They rarely suffer complications. Perhaps the sitting position is more physiologic, minimizing obstetric trauma; the Chinese have used this position for centuries. Maybe we bright young physicians could learn something.

Delivery of the infant will occur whether the obstetrician is present or still speeding to the hospital. Of course, no experienced obstetric nurse would ever try to restrain the baby's emerging head. If the mother is bleeding, draw blood for tests and cross-matching; start an intravenous infusion of saline; and resist the urge to investigate the cervix in the examination room.

Obstetric forceps hold a life between the blades. Properly used, elective outlet forceps can materially shorten the final stage of labor, but in inexperienced hands, permanent damage to the infant can result. The malar ecchymosis following forceps delivery of the infant is of no consequence and should be pointed out to the mother only to reassure her.

The episiotomy is a vital part of the delivery of all but the most flaccid multiparas. That little cut, allowing speedy safe delivery of the infant without vaginal tearing is what the patient pays her doctor for. Indeed, the episiotomy is a small sacrifice to the cause of youthful responsive vaginal tone in years to come.

Shaking chills sometimes follow delivery, usually related to a little amniotic fluid leaking into the blood stream. No therapy is necessary, and the chills usually subside promptly.

The 6-week check-up terminates the routine care of pregnancy. Ask your patient, "Does it hurt when you have sexual relations?" Of course, you told her not to, but most patients will give a definite yes or no response. Check the vaginal tone, the true test of your episiotomy; examine the cervix and fundus. Finally, discuss birth control and your patient's plans for future children. After all, pregnancy should be more than a failure of contraception.

References and Suggestions for Further Reading

1. Behrman S J, Kistner R W: Progress in Infertility. Boston, Little, Brown, 1968.
2. Benson R C: Handbook of Obstetrics and Gynecology. Los Altos, Calif, Lange, 1968.
3. Brant H A, Lachelin G C L: Vibration of cervix to expedite first stage of labor. Lancet 2:686–688, 1971.
4. Burch J C, Byrd B F Jr: Effects of long-term administration of estrogen on occurrence of mammary cancer in women. Ann Surg 174:414–417, 1971.
5. Calderone M S: Manual of Family Planning and Contraceptive Practice. Baltimore, Williams & Wilkins, 1970.
6. Drill V A: Oral Contraceptives. New York, McGraw-Hill, 1966.
7. Ford C V, Atkinson R M, Bragonier J R: Therapeutic abortion: Who needs a psychiatrist? Obstet Gynecol 38:206–213, 1971.
8. Janovski N A: Color Atlas of Gross Gynecologic and Obstetric Pathology. New York, McGraw-Hill, 1969.
9. Kistner R W: Gynecology: Principles and Practice. Chicago, Year Book, 1971.
10. McDonald R L: The role of emotional factors in obstetric complications. Psychosom Med 30:222–237, 1968.
11. Novak E R, Jones G S, Jones H W Jr: Gynecology. Baltimore, Williams & Wilkins, 1971.
12. Rheingold J C: The Fear of Being a Woman. New York, Grune & Stratton, 1964.
13. Rickels K, Garcia C-R, Fisher E: A measure of emotional distress in private gynecologic practice. Obstet Gynecol 38:139–146, 1971.
14. Shettles L B: Use of the Y chromosome in prenatal sex determination. Nature 230:-52–53, 1971.
15. Tindall V R: Dysmenorrhoea. Br Med J 1:329–331, 1971.
16. Willson J R, Beecham C T, Carrington E R: Obstetrics and Gynecology. St Louis, Mosby, 1966.

10

Genial Geriatrics

To be seventy years old . . . is like climbing the Alps. You reach a snow-crowned summit, and see behind you the deep valley stretching miles and miles away, and before you other summits higher and whiter, which you may have strength to climb, or may not. Then you sit down and meditate and wonder which it will be.

Henry Wadsworth Longfellow
(1807–1882)

Geriatric medicine is as much a specialty as pediatrics; it is the study of diseases peculiar to an age of man. With ever-growing legions of citizens marching past the sixty-fifth milestone, and with the current trend toward increased specialization in medicine, I look for geriatrics to become a respected medical specialty within the next two decades, with a certifying board, diplomas, and other trappings of the traditional medical disciplines.

The geriatric age can be indoor winter loneliness. The geriatrician needs a firm knowledge of the degenerative diseases and compassion for the problems of the elderly—the relentless pain of worn-out joints, the inability to hear a favorite concerto, the caprice of recent memory, the indignity of chronic constipation, and the grief of watching contemporaries, one by one, lose their race with time.

DEALING WITH THE GERIATRIC PATIENT

Dignity is a right of the senior citizen. Address your elderly patient as Mrs. Jones or Mr. Smith. Your 82-year-old patient was born in the last century and reared in an age of stiff collars and stiffer customs, when young adults addressed their elders by Christian name only as a sign of disrespect and in peril of a severe thrashing. Calling retired Mr. John Smith "Johnny" is disrespectful, undignified, and inexcusable.

Oldsters are often cantankerous. Santiago Ramón y Cajal (1852–1934) remarked: "It is idle to dispute with old men. Their opinions, like their cranial sutures, are ossified."

Learn to roll with the punches. Much of your oldster's medical folklore has historical basis in fact and should be supplemented, not bludgeoned, by modern medicine. When 88-year-old Mrs. Green refuses to have a lump in her breast removed, she may be showing better judgment than her physician, and old Mr. Johnson's constipation may well respond to hot water and lemon juice, aided by some Metamucil each day.

Deafness can cloud communication, your hoarse shouting interrupted by hearing-aid feedback. Try placing your stethoscope in the patient's ears and speaking into the bell (Fig. 10–1). He will probably hear you clearly. The stethoscope is an effective hearing aid, reminiscent of the old ear trumpet.

Hospitalization terrifies the geriatric patient, who recalls bygone days when hospitals were for dying. Frightened when he enters, the elderly patient leaves his familiar home and handy landmarks to be interred in a strange bed and surrounded by alien white-robed beings. Is it any wonder that, when the lights go off at night, confusion begins? The night nurse promptly solves the geriatric patient's nocturnal confusion by shackling his arms to the bedrails. Be compassionate. When possible, treat your patient at home with house calls supplemented by telephone reports.

PROBLEMS OF THE GERIATRIC PATIENT

Insomnia plagues oldsters, often related to physical inactivity and emotional impoverishment. In 1907, Elbert G. Hubbard observed: "Insomnia never comes to a man who has to get up exactly at six o'clock. Insomnia troubles only those who can sleep any time." Beware the afternoon napper; he isn't sleepy at bedtime and comes to you request-

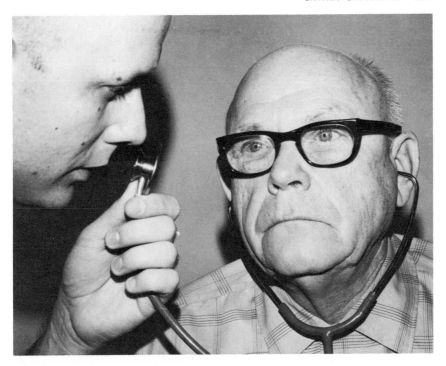

Fig. 10–1. Use your stethoscope as a hearing aid when you talk to a hard-of-hearing patient.

ing sleeping pills. Instead, prescribe a specific bedtime, an hour of arising, followed by purposeful activity during the day. Get him out of the house whenever possible. Involve him in church work and a local Senior Citizens' Club. Prescribe sedation only as a last resort.

Loss of appetite may be due to physical inactivity or may signal depression in the elderly. Certainly, a multivitamin supplement is indicated. A small glass of wine may spark mealtime. As Maimonides wrote in the twelfth century Mishna Torah: "Honey and wine are bad for children but salutary for the elderly." A little spiritus frumenti is a good tonic.

Medication dosage in geriatrics, as in pediatrics, must be tailored to the patient's age, weight, and activity. The standard dose of belladonna may relieve your patient's gastritis, but lead to oppressive constipation or urinary retention. Digitalis intoxication is common in elderly patients, and diuretics can cause marked lethargy, with or without excessive potassium loss.

Sedatives are treacherous in the elderly: Barbiturates often lead to confusion and mania by depressing higher centers in the brain. Chloral hydrate, the old-fashioned Mickey Finn, is the best all-around bedtime sedation for the elderly; it is available in capsules or liquid. For sedation of the agitated patient, chlorpromazine (Thorazine) is good, but mesoridazine (Serentil) is often better, an initial intramuscular dosage of 25 mg providing smoother sedation with less depression. For a patient who resists Thorazine, Serentil, and Sparine in huge doses, try 0.5 mg of scopolamine intramuscularly, a safe smooth sedative for the agitated elderly patient.

The **Colostomy**, a vexing problem for the patient and the physician involved in its care, is an artificial anus lacking the sphincter muscle. Unless controlled by daily irrigation, the colostomy will discharge feces at capricious times. Colostomy irrigation, like the low enema, initiates peristalic action without mechanically flushing the bowel clean. Instruct your patient in the technique of colostomy irrigation as follows: The patient sits straddling the toilet, facing the tank. He attaches an 18-inch plastic drainage sheath to a colostomy ring held in place by an elastic belt. The sheath is used to direct the flow into the toilet. Astride the toilet with the drainage sheath in place, he cuts a small opening in the plastic sheath near the stoma, allowing the introduction of the syringe tip into the colostomy. He fills with warm water an 8-oz rubber bulb syringe with a flexible tip, lubricates the tip, and inserts it through the hole in the drainage sheath into the colostomy to a depth of about 4 inches. With gentle pressure, he empties the syringe. He repeats the process two or three times, using 16 to 24 oz of water. After the syringe tip is removed, the colostomy will drain water and feces down the sheath into the toilet; this will be followed by a bowel movement under peristaltic stimulation. Once irrigation is completed, a standard colostomy bag is worn for about 30 minutes, following which the stoma need be covered only with a 4-inch by 4-inch gauze pad.

Bedsores represent a failure of nursing care and are preventable. Sustained pressure over a bony prominence, particularly if soaked in urine or feces, rapidly leads to ulceration of the skin. Once established, bedsores strongly resist therapy, eventually yielding after months of struggle. Prevent bedsores by instructing the nurse to turn your bedfast patient from side to back to side every 2 hours day and night. A sheepskin pad under the buttocks minimizes pressure and provides ventilation; a water bed or circulating air mattress are useful aids, but the best prophylaxis against bedsores remains frequent changing of the patient's position. To prevent is better than to heal.

Turning the patient in bed to examine his back is a common cause of that occupational hazard of physicians—the low back strain. Foolishly bending forward from the waist, the physician lifts and pushes, exerting tremendous leverage on his own low back muscles. Turn the bedfast patient as follows: Elevate the bed to its maximum height, and walk to the side of the bed the patient will face when turned. Bring the patient's opposite arm and leg toward you as far as possible, rolling the shoulder and hip as they move (Fig. 10–2). Once the arm and leg are positioned, much of the patient's weight has been turned and a slow steady pull on the hip and shoulder completes the maneuver, smoothly turning the patient in bed to face you.

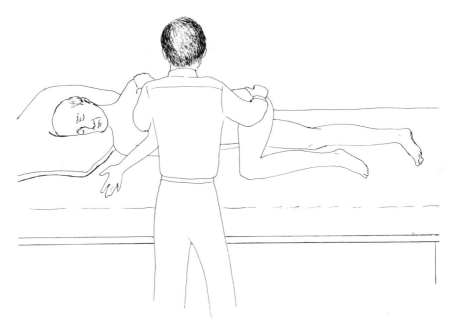

Fig. 10–2. To turn a patient in bed, turn his shoulder and hip first.

Tube feeding through a nasogastric tube can sustain the comatose elderly patient long after all superficial veins have been exhausted. The tube should be inserted, the feeding administered, and the tube removed. Never leave a feeding tube taped in place; excessive secretions can cause pneumonia. And never tape the tube so it exerts pressure against the soft nasal ala, lest you and your patient be punished with a disfiguring deep ulceration. A twice daily tube feeding, containing nothing more than a homogenized geriatric diet plus milk and pulverized medication, will sustain your elderly comatose patient until he recovers.

Vaginal examination of the geriatric patient is often neglected on grounds of technical difficulty. It should not be. The 86-year-old patient with vaginal bleeding can be afforded the benefit of pelvic examination without leaving her bed. Cover an inverted bedpan with a sheet and place it under her buttocks, elevating the introitus to an accessible position (Fig. 10–3). Her knees are bent and her legs held in place by nurses. With the patient in this position, your $500 examination table offers no greater convenience.

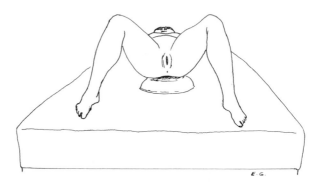

Fig. 10–3. Position a bedfast patient for a pelvic examination by elevating her hips on an inverted bedpan.

GERIATRIC REHABILITATION

Rehabilitation is a major goal of geriatric medicine, especially important following a stroke or a hip fracture. Begin at the moment of the original insult. A footboard at the end of the bed prevents extension contractures of the ankle caused by the weight of bedsheets. Between passive exercises, a paralyzed arm may be held in place with a sling and at other times positioned fully extended at the side or up along the head. A rolled wash cloth in the hand minimizes flexion contractures of the fingers, and a sandbag or a pillow beside the foot prevents external rotation contracture of the hip.

Passive exercises should begin as soon as the acute phase of the stroke has waned. An intelligent family member or a nurse's aide can do a creditable job, once she understands the principle; every involved joint must be passively moved through its full range of motion several times daily—every finger, every toe, wrist, elbow, shoulder, hip, knee, and ankle. Look for full extension and full flexion as each joint is moved.

Inactive elderly joints develop contractures as fast as you can say "physical therapy," and anticipation must be the watchword.

Active exercises presume voluntary muscular motion and supplement passive exercise of the joints. The rubber ball in the hand, the weight on a pulley, and moving against the resistance of the therapist's hand are time-honored methods. When possible, increase coordination by insisting that your patient use his paralyzed side to eat his meals, button his shirt, and comb his hair. Encourage family members to engage him in card games or chess to improve manual dexterity on the involved side.

Weight-lifting increases muscle tone. An ordinary steam iron or a single volume of the household encyclopedia weighing 4 or 5 lb will do.

Encouragement overcomes apathy. Push your patient to get moving. As rapidly as possible, have him sit in bed, then in a chair, then stand next to the bed. Using parallel bars gives him a sense of accomplishment; then graduate him to a walker or crutches. Supervise the therapy yourself; it is just as important as pinning the hip or saving the patient's life during the acute phase of his stroke. Give your patient confidence; his goal is independent walking out the hospital door and home.

THE NURSING HOME

Nursing homes are a booming industry, filling a need created by millions of senior citizens who have outlived their cerebral circulation. At present, there are more than 23,000 nursing homes in the United States, containing more than 1 million patient beds. Some nursing homes are better than others, and Medicare certification is a rough guide to the facilities and level of care provided.

Is a nursing home needed? As many have discovered to their sorrow, Medicare does not automatically approve the admission of every senior citizen to a nursing home. An application for extended care benefits will be categorically disallowed unless all the following criteria are met:

1. The condition must require continuing skilled nursing care.
2. The physician must certify and order the specific continuing skilled nursing care needed.
3. The patient must have been in a qualified hospital for at least 3 consecutive days before admission to the extended care facility.

4. The patient must be admitted to the extended care facility within 14 days after leaving the hospital.

5. Treatment at the extended care facility must be a continuation of therapy of the illness for which the patient was hospitalized.

"Continuing skilled nursing care" is a sneaky phrase, resulting in disallowal of thousands of extended care requests annually, many because the attending physician failed to study the criteria for acceptability. Do *not* assume that your patient's nursing home sojourn will be smiled upon by Medicare merely because the following services are provided: dressing changes, colostomy care, bedsore treatment, massage, heat treatments, whirlpool therapy, range-of-motion exercises, gait training, oxygen therapy "as necessary," sporadic injections, indwelling catheter maintenance.

Indwelling catheter?! That's right. Here's an example of the legerdemain practiced by those friendly clerks at your regional Medicare intermediary: An indwelling catheter used as an adjunct to active disease of the urinary tract may require continuous skilled nursing care, but the same indwelling catheter necessary because of incontinence does not require special care, other than changing at weekly intervals, and the patient is not entitled to extended care benefits.

Rules change faster than textbooks go to press, but the moral of the story remains. When your patient applies for benefits from the government—be it federal, state, or local—he counts upon you to assist him knowledgeably in attaining his legislated benefits. Doctor, beside knowing medicine, you've got to know the law.

Extended care benefits, once approved, usually fail to cover all nursing home costs. Medicare spokesmen have promulgated misconceptions that result in bitter disappointment once the patient discovers the facts. If you recommend an extended care facility, let your patient know from the beginning what he can expect from Medicare while in the nursing home: Part A of Medicare helps pay for:

1. A semiprivate bed and meals, including special diets
2. Regular nursing services provided by the extended care facility
3. Drugs administered by the extended care facility
4. Occupational, physical, and speech therapy
5. Medical supplies and appliances, including casts, splints, braces, and wheelchairs
6. Medical social services

While the patient is in an extended care facility, Part A of Medicare does *not* pay for:

1. Personal convenience items, such as television or private telephone
2. Private-duty nurses
3. Physicians' fees
4. The extra charge for a private room unless certified as medically necessary

Extended care benefits are completely covered up to a variable dollar maximum for the first 20 days; another 80 days of care are covered except for $8.50 a day, which the patient must pay. When the Medicare intermediary determines that the maximum benefit of extended care has been reached, Part A coverage will be terminated.

If you don't agree with Medicare's denial of extended care benefits for your patient, you owe it to him to request reconsideration. A sincere impassioned plea won't do. You must fulfill all the necessary criteria and outline a medically necessary, specifically prescribed, course of treatment requiring continuous skilled nursing care expected to result in substantial improvement or rehabilitation of your patient. In practice, daily physical therapy is your best bet, most applicable in cases of stroke or hip fracture. Many appeals can be avoided by careful attention to the original Medicare certification of your extended care patient.

References and Suggestions for Further Reading

1. Anderson W F: Practical Management of the Elderly. Philadelphia, Davis, 1971.
2. Astrand P O: Physical performance as a function of age. JAMA 205:729–733, 1968.
3. Cowdry E V: The Care of the Geriatric Patient, 3rd ed. St Louis, Mosby, 1968.
4. Ewy G A, Marcus F I: Digitalis therapy in the aged. Am Fam Physician GP 1:81–85, 1970.
5. Freeman J T: Physicians and long-term care facilities. J Am Geriatr Soc 19:847–859, 1971.
6. Human Aging: A Biological and Behavioral Study. Public Health Service Publication No 986. Washington, DC, US Dept Health, Education, Welfare, 1963.
7. Lowenthal M F, Zilli A: Colloquium on Health and Aging of the Population. Basel, Karger, 1969.
8. O'Malley K: Effect of age and sex on human drug metabolism. Br Med J 3:607–609, 1971.
9. Rossman I: Clinical Geriatrics. Philadelphia, Lippincott, 1971.
10. Rudd J L, Margolin R J: Maintenance Therapy for the Geriatric Patient. Springfield, Ill, Thomas, 1968.

11. Saunders G A: Myocardial infarction in elderly surgical patient. Geriatrics 26:122–128, 1971.

12. Taylor R B: Games Medicare people play. Physician's Management 11:56–57, 1971.

13. Wilkins E G: Constipation in the elderly. Postgrad Med 44:728–732, 1968.

11

Sane Psychiatry

If a patient is poor he is committed to a public hospital as "psychotic;" if he can afford the luxury of a private sanitarium, he is put there with the diagnosis of "neurasthenia;" if he is wealthy enough to be isolated in his own home under constant watch of nurses and physicians he is simply an indisposed "eccentric."

Pierre Marie Felix Janet
(1859–1947)

Twenty-three centuries ago Hippocrates described mental illness and chronic brain disease, admonishing fledgling physicians to treat their patients gently. Not so during the Middle Ages; then the mentally ill were considered to be under Satan's influence, and to "cure" them the Devil was exorcised with fiendish maneuvers. In the early sixteenth century, Paracelsus ascribed psychotic behavior to astrologic influences, and in 1547, King Henry VIII chartered the Hospital of St. Mary of Bethlehem (commonly know as Bedlam); there the mentally deranged were "treated" with shackles and chains, and the word "bedlam" achieved a niche in the English vocabulary as a synonym for madhouse. In the early nineteenth century, Mesmer described his theories of animal magnetism, and the work of Charcot in Paris paved the way for the later schools of Adler, Jung, and Freud—the putative fathers of modern psychiatry.

OFFICE PSYCHIATRY

If you believe the statistics, 1 of every 20 Americans suffers from mental illness. Some days I think they have all gathered in my waiting room. Certainly, not all are psychotic; many suffer from disabling anxiety, hyperventilation, cancerophobia, reactive depression, and marital unrest.

The vanguard of psychiatry is the office practitioner, spearheading modern medicine's attack upon the collective neuroses of an anxious world. The mindless referral of all emotional illness to the psychiatrist would soon demolish the specialist's schedule and swamp the available resources.

Office psychiatry takes time, considerably more minutes than are needed to deal with the average wart, burn, or ear infection. The initial interview will be the longest; later visits demand less time. When shoehorning these patients into a crowded schedule, try this tip: Schedule the lengthy psychiatric interview at the end of the morning or afternoon office hours, and send your staff home for lunch or dinner. By this scheduling ploy, you are not paying your staff to sit idly through a long interview, and other patients are not forming a log jam in the waiting room. The quick lunch or delayed dinner is a small price for an orderly office schedule that day, and if the patient gets hungry, that helps wind up the interview.

Through the window of my consultation room, the noon-hour conference patient can view the parking lot and observe the arrival of the 1 P.M. patients; this too helps bring the session to a close.

Fatigue spares no age group from pediatrics to geriatrics and is usually, but not always, of psychiatric origin. Ask the patient, "Do you wake up tired in the morning or wear out during the day?" The anxious depressed patient arises with the blahs, drags his weary bones from bed, and faces the day with all the enthusiasm of a condemned criminal. The man who awakens refreshed after 8 hours of sleep and then poops out at 11 A.M. may, indeed, suffer from organic illness, such as anemia, leukemia, or hypoglycemia.

Responsibility is a heavy weight to bear, grinding many good men into submission. As the story goes, your patient, John Smith, functioned well as a machinist and later as a shop foreman, but when his productivity was rewarded by a promotion to assistant manager, John promptly developed insomnia, gastritis, and fatigue. He used to work 12 hours at his drill press and then go bowling that evening, but now the burden of responsibility is too heavy. Your best advice to John: Reject the promotion and stay healthy.

Arbitrating **marital conflicts** is like the Vietnam peace talks—time-consuming, frustrating, and likely doomed to failure. Enter the fray only if both camps agree to negotiations. Then hear both sides; find out what the fight is really about. Is there a focal problem of infidelity or physical abuse? Or have these two persons who once pledged their troth for better or worse evolved a sick relationship of innuendo and bickering?

Have each spouse write a list of the other's most intolerable actions, the worst first. When these lists are handed in, put them away and ask each spouse for another list—this time of his *own* most serious marital shortcomings. Then compare the lists and discuss them with the embattled couple. The tabulation can be revealing indeed.

Arbitrate a settlement to the marital conflict, laying down strict guidelines, in writing if necessary. Arguments must remain confined to the subject; no personal invective allowed. It will take weeks to establish lines of communication between these two people, who have probably spent the last few years in a dialogue of hate propaganda.

THE PSYCHIATRIC INTERVIEW

The psychiatric interview breaks away from the traditional history-examination-diagnosis-treatment medical consultation. Rather, it is a free-flowing interview involving a sympathetic exchange of ideas that brings out hidden facts and helps the patient gain insight.

G. K. Chesterton (1874–1936) quipped: "Psychoanalysis is confession without absolution." Right. The physician can give no one absolution, but he can help the patient to achieve insight into the nature of his problem.

Words are the scalpel and suture of psychiatry. Just as a television interviewer always has a few stock questions to pop to his celebrity guest when conversation palls ("if you were stranded on a desert island and could choose . . ."), you should have some stock questions to speed a lagging interview and keep the patient talking. Ask him: "If you had three wishes, what would they be?" "Are you doing what you want with your life?" "How do you feel about your problems?" "What single thing could you do to make your life more rewarding?"

Your patient has a job, a home, and a family; he doesn't live in your office, and when you interview him, he is in your environment, not his. Harvey Cushing (1869–1939) observed: "A physician is obligated to consider more than a diseased organ, more even than the whole man —he must view the man in his world." You will understand your patient's emotional problems only when you know the details of his home, family, hobbies, religion, and occupation.

Religion plays a larger role in mental illness than your patient may freely admit. Oppressive Catholicism and Baptist Fundamentalism leave their mark on the growing child. Portnoy stated the case against the Jewish mother. Unite these strains in matrimony, and the couple suffers a cultural schism while their offspring lacks ethnic identity.

Family attitudes color the mental picture. "How does your husband feel about your problems?" "Is he sympathetic?" "Does he seem to reject you?" "Do you unconsciously make things worse?" "Would the family like to come and talk with us next time?"

Crying frequently punctuates the psychiatric interview. What to do when the lady sobs uncontrollably? Do nothing; that cry is excellent therapy. Hand her your box of tissues and sit back. The crying won't last long, and your interview will be all the better for it.

PSYCHIATRIC THERAPY

Ventilation is the cornerstone of office psychiatric therapy, recognized instinctively by the patient searching for "someone to talk to." Except for directing the interview with questions, the physician remains passive. Keep your analysis to a minimum; coax the facts out of your patient and he will soon see the pattern. Shore up his sagging ego and help patch the pieces of his life together, but avoid the sticky overdependent relationship—the patient who won't cross the street without benefit of medical consultation.

Environmental change is valid psychotherapeutic technique. Many shaky egos function tolerably well day by day, until sidetracked by an environmental roadblock—a financial crisis, a death in the family, or the acquisition of an indwelling mother-in-law. Keep your eye on self-employed businessmen and shopkeepers; they "can't afford" to take vacations, but often end up spending that extra money on doctors' bills. Waning vitality may follow moonlighting, and the working mother really holds two jobs. Your patient's symptoms may respond to no deeper therapy than chucking the second job, finding a nice boarding home for mother-in-law, or indulging in a 2-week vacation. Many harried housewives have nothing that a maid, a million dollars, and a trip to Europe wouldn't cure.

Drug therapy plays an adjunctive role in office psychotherapy. A "nerve pill" won't solve your patient's problems, but it helps. Which tranquilizer should you prescribe? The overwhelming majority of your patients will respond to the minor tranquilizers—oxazepam (Serax), diazepam (Valium), or chlordiazepoxide (Librium). My personal favorite is Serax, available in 10-, 15-, and 30-mg capsules, usually prescribed in an initial dose of 15 mg three times daily. Ataxia has been described in patients taking Librium and Valium, but not Serax. Not effective in the usual dosage? Then consider higher doses of the minor tranquilizers before using the big guns.

The phenothiazines are major tranquilizers, indispensable in the treatment of major psychoses. Chlorpromazine (Thorazine), an excellent drug for the psychotic patient, is usually initiated in a dose of 25 mg three or four times daily, increased as necessary to control symptoms. If you think your patient needs Thorazine, perhaps he also needs a psychiatrist.

Depression is the target of a host of psychotropic agents. Amitriptyline (Elavil) and imipramine (Tofranil) share a usual starting dose of 25 mg three times daily, mild sedative properties, and a lag of several days before the full effect is seen. Doxepin (Sinequan), prescribed initially in a dose of 25 mg three or four times daily, is effective against anxiety associated with depression. Protriptyline (Vivactil), usually initiated as one 5-mg tablet three times daily, increases psychomotor activity and is useful in the fatigued, apathetic, depressed patient.

The tranquilizer-dependent patient can't cope with the world. Without her tranquilizer shield, she is shaky, disorganized, and vulnerable and totters on the brink of institutionalization. Short-circuited by sedatives, she can function—not a sparkling personality, but neither a liability for the family.

But she may overdo it. Pop a happy pill and she feels good; with two she feels better, and soon her prescription is gone. "Doctor, I'm sorry to bother you, but I spilled all my tranquilizers in the toilet bowl. Could you phone in another prescription?" Refuse and she'll turn to alcohol or worse. Give the prescription to another family member for safekeeping and, sooner or later, she'll find it.

What to do? Recognize the patient's need for tranquilizers; without them, she'll disintegrate. But underscore the dangers of overuse, reinforce her fragile ego, and put her on her honor, prescribing exactly enough medication to last until her next visit, a day or two later. Insist that there will be no repeat prescriptions and tell her to "take good care of those pills. Make them last." If this approach proves successful, schedule subsequent visits at increasingly long intervals, eventually attaining a maximum of once every month or two.

You will probably never be able to free this patient from her drug-dependence, and she should never be trusted with a refillable prescription for tranquilizers.

Reserpine deserves special mention. Used for centuries in Hindu medicine for the treatment of hypertension, mental illness, and insomnia, *Rauwolfia* came into vogue as an antihypertensive medication around 1955. Jubilant at the prospect of an effective specific hypotensive agent, physicians boarded the bandwagon of reserpine therapy.

Over the years, particularly before the newer, more potent antihypertensive medications were discovered, I prescribed reserpine for many patients with high blood pressure. Time passed, and sooner or later, almost every one of those patients has come to my office complaining of depression and fatigue—symptoms that vanished dramatically when reserpine was discontinued.

SUICIDE

The thought of suicide is a great consolation: by means of it one gets successfully through many a bad night.

Friedrich Nietzsche
(1844–1900)

The potential suicide victim has considered his case, judged himself unworthy, sentenced the defendant to death, and is about to act as executioner. Certainly, the patient is at the bottom of the valley of depression, convinced that escape is impossible or just not worth the effort.

Anger and depression consume the suicidal victim. Suicide is often the final and ultimate act of revenge. Although not "reasonable" by rational standards, to the victim, suicide seems the only proper solution to his problems.

The suicidal patient in the office presents a medical and medicolegal dilemma. He's depressed, apathetic, angry at the world or at some one. But will he attempt suicide? Would he really do it? Can he be trusted with medication? Or should you assert your authority and commit him to an institution?

Discuss the possibility of suicide with your patient. Find out if self-destruction has been considered; it probably has. "You seem pretty down in the dumps. What do you think you might do about it?"

Can the case be handled in the office? If your interview is fruitful, the patient's symptoms seem improved, and the likelihood of suicide seems lessened, he can probably be managed without institutionalization. Extract two promises from your patient: (1) a specific promise that he will not attempt suicide and (2) a promise that he will call you if suicidal temptations beckon. Then make sure another family member understands the arrangements; confirm that your patient won't be left alone, and schedule a specific revisit time for tomorrow.

Then stay available. The patient who has promised to call his physician when suicidal thoughts prevail will almost always keep his promise. Be there! A recording or, what's worse, an answering service cretin, can trigger a successful suicide. You must keep in touch with this patient until the crisis is resolved, even if it means giving him a theater or dinner party telephone number.

THE PSYCHIATRIC REFERRAL

When ventilation fizzles, drug therapy falters, environmental changes backfire, and your patient suspects a wiretap on his telephone line or an international conspiracy against him, and acquires an armory for self-protection, it is time for a psychiatric referral.

The psychiatric referral is a touchy business. As Walter Lincoln Palmer said: "Don't refer a patient to a psychiatrist as if you are telling him to go to hell." Never, never insult your patient's intelligence with subterfuge and don't compromise his trust by attempted deception.

The psychiatrist is a specialist who treats emotional problems. "Certainly, you wouldn't hesitate to consult a surgeon for appendicitis or a cardiologist for a heart attack. Now you have an emotional problem and we want the best help available. That's a psychiatrist. I'll be happy to make all the arrangements."

Is he reluctant?

Be logical but insistent. "A normal person doesn't record telephone conversations, shout obscenities at the doctor, walk around outdoors without his clothes on [or whatever the case may be]. Try to see yourself as you appear to others. You must have help. Now let's work together to arrange it."

Still refuses?

Use your paternal image to insist that the patient see the psychiatrist. Bully him verbally. And, as if talking with a child, state your orders as though you *expect* them to be obeyed. They usually will be.

The psychiatrist is not a magician. Don't promise miracles on the first visit. "If only we can get your wife to the psychiatrist!" It's not that easy, and you know it. The psychiatric referral is the first step up on the long hard climb to a normal psyche.

PSYCHIATRIC TERMS

The jargon of psychiatry is a specialized vocabulary, seldom heard in the general office. But when referring a patient to a specialist or institution, you have to know the words; vague descriptions won't do. The following is a glossary of selected psychiatric terms:

Abreaction. Free expression of repressed ideas and affect under psychotherapeutic influence

Acting out. Unconscious emotional conflicts expressed in symbolic actions, often socially unacceptable

Affective psychosis. Psychotic behavior marked by wide swings of mood

Anaclitic. Excessive dependence, as a child upon a parent, with symptoms developing upon separation

Association, clang. Nonsensical sound association or rhyming, sometimes seen in manic psychoses

Astasia-abasia. Lack of ability to stand or walk without demonstrable neuropathology, usually caused by hysteria

Automatism. Repetitious symbolic behavior often seen in schizophrenia

Bulimia. Pathologically increased hunger

Camptocormia. Neurotic hysterical forward body flexion

Catalepsy. Muscle rigidity and fixed posture, seen in schizophrenia and hysteria

Compulsion. A symbolic act performed in ritual fashion in spite of conscious efforts at avoidance

Confabulation. The imaginative manufacture of fantastic details to fill memory gaps, characteristic of alcoholic psychoses

Dereistic. Delusional thinking, without reference to reality

Displacement. The transfer of symbolic significance from one concept or object to another

Echolalia. Repetitive imitation of another's speech, seen in schizophrenia

Echopraxia. Repetitive imitation of another's movements, seen in schizophrenia

Fugue. A hysterical dissociation of the patient's consciousness and behavior

Hebephrenia. A type of schizophrenia with delusions, hallucinations, and silly behavior

Ideas of reference. Delusions that the patient is influenced by others, seen in paranoia

Introjection. Incorporation into the patient's ego of qualities of an object or another person

Obsession. A recurrent thought, recognized by the patient as irrational, compelling compulsive activity to relieve anxiety

Regression. Return to previously learned modes of behavior, often infantile

Repression. Unconscious banishing of ideas and desires to the subconscious

Stereotypy. Repetition of behavior or speech, seen in schizophrenia

Sublimation. Directing desires into socially acceptable activity

Suppression. Conscious banishing of impulses and ideas to the unconscious

RECOGNITION OF PSYCHIATRIC SYNDROMES

Symptom complexes characterize each psychiatric disorder, and knowledge of them allows accurate diagnosis and classification. The preparation of legal reports or commitment papers requires specific documentation of symptoms, supporting the final diagnosis. Sure, you can describe your specific observations of wild hostile behavior, perhaps aggressive, perhaps confused, but can you list the patient's symptoms in the proper psychiatric terms? The following outline should help:

Anxiety neuroses
    Anxiousness
    Hyperventilation
    Restlessness
    Rapid pulse
    Mild tremor of the fingers
    Exaggerated tendon reflexes

Delirium
    Clouded sensorium
    Delusions

    Distractibility
    Affect fearful
    Perceptual disturbances
    Rapid pulse
    Dilated pupils
    Diaphoresis
    Facial flushing

Depression
    Depressed mood
    Decreased motor activity
    Thought content pessimistic
    Impaired abstract judgment
    Nihilistic delusions
    Neglected personal appearance
    Possible weight loss
    Constipation

Mania
    Elated mood
    Increased motor activity
    Flight of ideas
    Fluctuating affect
    Frequent delusions
    Impaired judgment

Psychopathic personality
    Poor social adjustment, including poor work record, arrests, and divorce
    Unable to profit by experience
    Blames misfortune on others
    Overly friendly
    Chronic alcoholism a frequent problem

Schizophrenia
    Affect inappropriate, often bland
    Impaired insight
    Thought processes fragmented
    Echolalia and echopraxia common
    Clang association may be noted
    Ideas of influence and reference common
    Somatic delusions

Visual or auditory hallucinations
Hebephrenia may be seen

Schizophrenia, paranoid
A form of schizophrenia with findings noted above, particularly delusions of influence and reference
Ideas of persecution, systematized delusional system, integrated but illogical
Affect distortion
Disintegration of behavior
Acting out ideas of persecution
Potentially dangerous

References and Suggestions for Further Reading

1.   Aldrich C K: An Introduction to Dynamic Psychiatry. New York, McGraw-Hill, 1966.

2.   Berger F M: Drugs and suicide in the United States. Clin Pharmacol Ther 8:219–223, 1967.

3.   Blinder M G: Differential diagnosis and treatment of depressive disorders. JAMA 195:8–12, 1966.

4.   Bromet E, Harrow M, Tucker G J: Factors related to short-term prognosis in schizophrenia and depression. Arch Gen Psychiatry 25:149–155, 1971.

5.   Dyrud J: Treatment of anxiety states. Arch Gen Psychiatry 25:298–305, 1971.

6.   Enelow A J, Adler L: Psychiatric skills and knowledge for the general practitioner. JAMA 189:91–96, 1964.

7.   Freedman A M, Kaplan H I: Comprehensive Textbook of Psychiatry. Baltimore, Williams & Wilkins, 1967.

8.   Halleck S L: Hysterical personality traits. Arch Gen Psychiatry 16:750–757, 1967.

9.   Haughton A B: Suicide prevention programs: The current scene. Am J Psychiatry 124:1692–1696, 1968.

10.   Havens L L: Recognition of suicidal risks through the psychologic examination. N Engl J Med 276:210–215, 1967.

11.   Hogary G E, Katz M M: Norms of adjustment and social behavior. Arch Gen Psychiatry 25:470–480, 1971.

12.   Lesse S: Anxiety: Its Components, Development, and Treatment, New York, Grune & Stratton, 1970.

13.   Lesse S: Masked depression: A diagnostic and therapeutic problem. Dis Nerv System 29:169–173, 1968.

14.   Mace D R: The physician and marital sexual problems. Med Aspects Human Sex 5:50–62, 1971.

15.   McHugh P R, Goodell H: Suicidal behavior. Arch Gen Psychiatry 25:456–464, 1971.

16.   Ornstein P H: What is and what is not psychotherapy? Dis Nerv System 29:118–123, 1968.

17. Rosenthal S H: Recognition of depression. Geriatrics 23:111–115, 1968.

18. Schuster C R, Thompson T: Self-administration of and behavioral dependence on drugs. Annu Rev Pharmacol 9:483–502, 1969.

19. Schwab J J, Brown J: Treating anxiety and depression. Postgrad Med 44:60–69, 1968.

20. Schwab J J, Brown J: Uses and abuses of psychiatric consultation. JAMA 205:65–68 1968.

21. Spitzer R L, Wilson P T: A guide to the American Psychiatric Association's new diagnostic nomenclature. Am J Psychiatry 124:1619–1629, 1968.

22. Visher J S: Trends in psychiatric treatment: A report of a private psychiatric practice. Am J Psychiatry 125:959–963, 1969.

23. Zabarenko R N, Merenstein J, Zabarenko L: Teaching psychological medicine in the family practice office. JAMA 218:392–396, 1971.

12

The Emergency That Wasn't on the Schedule

Let me conduct you to the bedside of Charles II: With a cry he fell. Dr. King, who, fortunately, happened to be present, bled him with a pocket knife. Fourteen physicians were quickly in attendance. They bled him more thoroughly; they scarified and cupped him; they shaved and blistered his head; they gave him an emetic, a clyster, and two pills. During the next eight days they "threw in" fifty-seven separate drugs; and toward the end, a cordial containing forty more. This availing nothing, they tried Goa stone, which was a calculus obtained from a species of Indian goat; and as a final remedy, the distillate of human skull. In the case report it is recorded that the emetic and the purge worked so mightily well that it was a wonder the patient died.

Sir Andrew MacPhail
British Medical Journal 1:445
1933

The physician's role in the drama of emergency is always a major one, sometimes calling for swift decisive action, but often demanding the more difficult quality of judicious restraint.

"Doctor, you've got to do something." And in the flush of excitement, you may oversedate the injured patient or further displace an unstable fracture.

The practicing physician is only a telephone call away from his next emergency. The community authority on the care of injuries, you are expected to direct on-the-spot treatment, splinting, and transportation of emergency patients. Tardiness, clumsiness, and lack of preparation can contribute to the patient's suffering and irrevocably tarnish your local image.

DEALING WITH EMERGENCIES

The emergency telephone call demands attention. "Doctor, something terrible has happened. You've got to come quickly." Find out what's going on. Whenever possible, get the patient on the phone; the caller may be a hysterical teenager reacting to a minor accident. Is the emergency a laceration which should be treated with compression and a fast trip to your office? Is it an injured ankle that should be x-rayed?

True emergencies requiring house calls occur daily—stroke, heart attack, and fractured hip. However inconvenient, these emergencies require immediate attention. The family at home with a patient suffering sudden hemiplegia or lying on the floor with a probable fractured hip has minimal interest in your busy schedule that afternoon or your dinner party that evening. You are needed at your patient's bedside. Now! Get in your car and go.

The doctor's **emergency bag** can spare you the embarrassment of arriving without the necessary instrument. Here is a list of items to keep in your black bag for emergencies:

1. A Resusitube plastic airway; the adult size will serve for children as young as 2 years of age
2. A tracheotomy set: three 13-gauge needles or one of those handy tracheotomy "pocket knives"
3. Bayonet forceps and nasal packing
4. Bandage scissors
5. A Kelly clamp
6. A 3-inch Ace bandage
7. A rectal examination glove and a small package of lubricating jelly
8. Silver nitrate applicator sticks
9. Emergency medications, including adrenalin, caffeine sodium benzoate, phenobarbital, injectable diazepam (Valium), injectable digoxin (Lanoxin), and meperidine (Demerol).

EMERGENCY CARE OF TRAUMATIC INJURIES

Ambrose Bierce (1842–1914?) described an accident as "an inevitable occurrence due to the action of immutable natural laws."

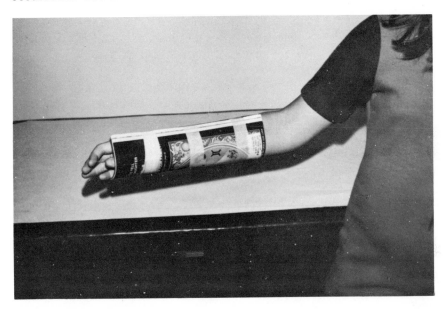

Fig. 12–1. The magazine splint.

The accident victim lies along the highway or at the foot of a ladder, surrounded by curious onlookers and, even worse, helpful first-aiders. Thank the first-aiders, dismiss the onlookers, and begin emergency therapy, considering the vital functions first.

Airway obstruction takes top priority; it is often relieved by simply rolling the patient on his side and cleaning out his mouth with your finger. If necessary, insert your Resusitube and carefully tape it in place. If indicated, a helper can maintain assisted ventilation.

Bleeding must be stopped—not the scant oozing from abrasions, but the pumping arterial blood loss from a deep laceration. Remove the tourniquet applied by some middle-aged boy scout; it is enhancing bleeding by increasing venous pressure. Then use 4-inch by 4-inch gauze pads to apply compression directly to the bleeding site, staunching the flow of blood.

Shock may be manifested as diaphoresis, tachycardia, and falling blood pressure. Until the patient can receive definitive therapy in the hospital, elevate his legs to increase venous return to the circulation and keep him warm. Allow fluids by mouth only if he is conscious.

Fractures and lacerations have low priority in the management of a trauma victim. They receive attention only after you have dealt with airway obstruction, bleeding, and shock. Cover lacerations with gauze pads and suture at your leisure. Attempt no reduction of fractures until the patient has been evaluated at the hospital, but splint all suspected bony injuries to minimize further trauma and pain.

Apply emergency splints over clothing without attempting definitive diagnosis at the accident site. Splint on suspicion, accepting the fracture position as found. Handle gently. Only a sadist tests for crepitus.

The magazine splint forms a handy cylinder, vastly superior to the traditional flat piece of wood (Fig. 12–1). Carry a few old magazines in the trunk of your car for use in emergencies. In the office, the emergency splint is as handy as that old *Newsweek* in your waiting room.

A pillow splint cushions the injured extremity and minimizes motion at the fracture site. A home injury can be effectively splinted with an ordinary bed pillow (Fig. 12–2), allowing painless transportation to the hospital for x-rays and evaluation.

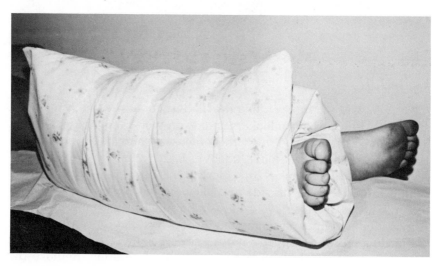

Fig. 12–2. The pillow splint.

Hidden internal bleeding must be considered in all victims of severe trauma. A lacerated liver can drip blood like a leaking faucet and a ruptured spleen gushes like a broken pipe. When a hip is fractured, up to two units of blood can be lost to the circulation without a single drop evident on the skin. In the sixteenth century, John Lyly observed: "The wound that bleedeth inward is most dangerous."

A **tension pneumothorax** is a mechanically efficient flutter valve. With each inspiration, more air enters the chest cavity, is trapped within the parietal pleura, and compromises lung function. Here is a roadside emergency where you can do more than join the crowd awaiting the ambulance: Put a finger in the dike. Occlude the opening with gauze pads or a clean handkerchief held or taped in place. Dramatically, the patient's respirations should improve.

The **flail chest** results from multiple rib fractures causing paradoxical respiration. Expansion of the chest sucks in the flail fragment with no more air movement than a lazy August day. Emergency stabilization of the flail chest is life-saving: Retract the fragment by attaching towel clips with counterweights for traction. Out along the road? No towel clips? Then stabilize the flail fragment with a bulky dressing taped securely in place, allowing inspiration of air upon chest expansion.

The **cervical spine injury** is an explosive problem with a short fuse; the disaster of paraplegia is an ever-present worry. Don't let a first-aid expert wiggle the victim's neck to see if it is broken. Before examining the neck, check peripheral motor and sensory function. Then gently percuss the top of the head (Fig. 12–3); if the cervical spine is fractured this procedure will elicit vociferous complaints. Of course, this patient must be moved only on a backboard with sandbags to stabilize the head. Remove a door from its hinges to improvise a backboard and fill two pillow cases with dirt to make emergency sandbags.

A **skull fracture** involving the wall of the frontal sinus occurs when the patient's moving head encounters a dashboard that has come to rest. The tip-off is crepitus of the eyelids caused by subcutaneous emphysema caused by air escaping from the frontal sinus.

EMERGENCIES CAUSED BY DRUGS

Drug experimentation is a growing problem, manifested in such insanities as drug-mixing parties, where each participant contributes a handful of pills, which are mixed in a salad bowl and passed around like candy. That's right. It really happens. And you will be called to treat the reactions.

Ups and downs—that's how kids classify drugs—with the simplicity of folklore and the familiarity of experience. And these are the two reactions you will face. The "up" reaction to mind-expanding drugs and the "down" reaction to narcotic depressants.

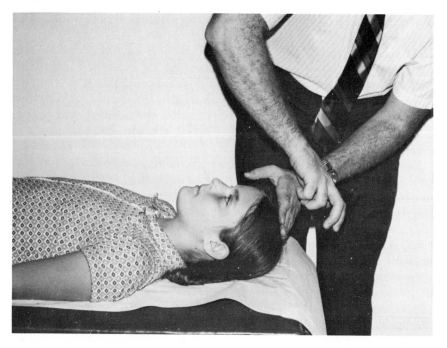

Fig. 12–3. Test for cervical spine injury by percussing the top of the head.

The **bad trip** is an up experience gone wild, the victim tilting madly with the windmills of his mind. The patient on a bummer may have taken one or more of the happy hallucinogens—LSD (D-lysergic acid diethylamide), peyote (mescaline), certain mushrooms (psilocybin), diethyltriptamine (DET), dimethyltriptamine (DMT), dimethyoxymethylamphetamine (DOM or STP), morning glory seeds *(Rivera corimbosa),* or methylene dioxyamphetamine (MDA or the love drug).

Talking down is accepted therapy of the bad trip, splinting the patient's shattered ego and relieving his panic and confusion. Take control of the situation; you must be in charge, offering support and reassurance. Keep your statements simple, direct, and repetitive. Confirm the patient's identity in relation to himself, the surroundings, and yourself. Help him reconstruct the familiar framework of reality by means of simple statements about persons present and objects in the room. Reassure him that the terrors of the mind are drug-induced and will pass. Tell him that his friends and family will continue to care for him. Be firm in your assertions. Repeat. Repeat.

Once underway, the therapy of a bad trip may be turned over to a narcotics case worker, your office nurse, or capable parents. Within a few hours, the symptoms will pass. Under no circumstances should the patient be left alone during a bad trip.

Narcotic overdosage, in an ironic sense, is often what the patient paid for. The "nickel bag" is usually cut with inert powder and contains a minimum of heroin. One day the addict gets his hands on a few full-strength bags, and about an hour later you are called to the bedside of a comatose youngster.

Treat narcotic overdosage with good nursing care, assisted ventilation if needed, and specific narcotic antagonists. Insert an airway; if respiratory depression threatens, the patient will require endotracheal intubation with assisted ventilation. Frequent position changes help prevent pneumonia, important because narcotics suppress the cough reflex. Airway suction may be necessary.

Narcotic antagonists help counteract the respiratory depression of narcotic overdosage but may not brighten your patient's state of consciousness. Nalorphine (Nalline) should be administered intravenously in a dose of 5 to 10 mg, repeated every 30 minutes as necessary. Also effective is levallorphan tartrate (Lorfan), 1 mg given intravenously as necessary.

Continued care of your flower child is a moral responsibility. The use of drugs is a symptom, not a disease. What is wrong in this youngster's life that compels him to turn to drugs? Solve the problems and drugs are discarded. Once the medical emergency is over, guide your patient into a local narcotics program or counseling service, and maybe you won't have to save his life again next month.

BITES, STINGS AND FISHHOOKS

Snake Bite emergency treatment prevents dissemination of the venom. Apply a tourniquet proximal to the bite and submerge the area in ice until definitive therapy with local excision, specific antivenom, and high-dosage corticosteroids can be undertaken.

Dog bites abound during warm summer months when active children annoy cranky canines. The bite is a tetanus-prone wound, and the victim requires prophylaxis against tetanus. Thorough scrubbing and surgical debridement are mandatory in all cases, followed by primary closure of selected facial wounds.

How about rabies vaccine? Find the animal and your troubles are over, of course. But the patient bitten by a bashful beast that eludes capture must be considered for rabies prophylaxis. Here's where your attention to state and county public health bulletins pays off. Is rabies common in your area, found in both wild and domestic animals? Then administer rabies vaccine if the animal remains at large. Live in a rabies-free area, the last case reported in a bat 4 years ago? Then explain to the family the remote likelihood of rabies and the real possibility of vaccine intoxication; most families will properly elect to forego rabies prophylaxis in these cases.

Insect stings cause many a "golf-course coronary." First aid of the insect sting, like the snake bite, involves a tourniquet and ice to delay absorption of toxins. Medical treatment includes the subcutaneous injection of 0.3 ml of 1:1000 aqueous adrenalin and the intramuscular or intravenous injection of 4 mg of dexamethasone (Decadron). Don't forget to continue the corticosteroid, tapering off slowly over the next week. Every patient with a proved allergy to stinging insects should receive desensitization injections and carry an adrenalin aerosol, such as Medihaler-Epi.

Ticks cling stubbornly to the skin of dogs, cattle, and humans. The tick usually releases his grasp when touched with the burning end of a cigarette. Farmers often use kerosene, gasoline, or turpentine on stubborn ticks. If the patient is brought to the office for treatment, you can usually grasp the tick near its mouth with hemostatic forceps and lift it gently from the skin. Thorough disinfection should follow. Avoid squeezing the body of the tick, injecting saliva and venom into the host's skin.

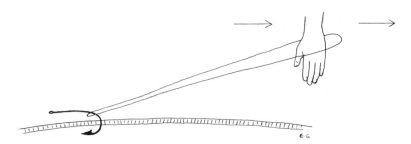

Fig. 12–4. Fisherman's method of hook removal.

Fishhook Removal in the office is easy, with lidocaine, scalpel, and forceps at the ready; but how about a fishhook injury on the boat or in the woods? Use the New England fishermen's method of removal (Fig. 12–4). Pass a loop of string or fishing line 20 to 30 inches long around the hook. Steady the base of the hook with one hand, and with the other hand, snap the loop of string sharply, releasing the fishhook.

THIS IS AN EMERGENCY

Healing is a matter of time, but it is sometimes also a matter of opportunity.

Hippocrates
(460–377 B.C.)

The **restaurant coronary** occurs as your medium-rare steak is placed in front of you. Across the room, a stranger gags, moans, grasps his chest, and falls to the floor. All eyes turn to you—the doctor on-the-spot. What to do?

Most restaurant coronaries, of course, are not coronaries at all, but airway occlusion by a bolus of food—the toll of gluttony.

If the airway is patent, emitting strident tones, but allowing adequate oxygenation, there is little to do. The gasping gourmand is best managed in the hospital. Stay at his side until the ambulance arrives.

But the obstruction is complete! Only swift decisive action can save your patient. If you have your curved Kelly clamp in your jacket pocket, extend the patient's neck, depress his tongue, and remove the bolus deftly. Left your Kelly clamp at home? Try to reach the obstructing morsel with your fingers; if that is unsuccessful, attempt to get the patient on all fours with his head dependent. Sometimes gravity, supplemented by a sharp blow between the shoulder blades, will dislodge the pellet.

All has failed. Within moments the patient becomes cyanotic and moribund. There's just one chance—an emergency tracheotomy.

Use the steak knife that came with your now-cold dinner. Following a rapid midline incision, feel for a tracheal ring with your finger and plunge in. Hold the airway open with a tube; the hollow barrel of a ballpoint pen is ideal (Fig. 12–5). Then call for help, see that your patient arrives safely at the hospital emergency room, and order another steak, medium rare.

Insulin reactions occurs when the diabetic injects his daily dose of insulin and neglects the meals that should follow. Sweating and shakiness are followed by confusion, which leads to coma if untreated. Brain damage due to hypoglycemia is a threat. In the early stages, insulin reaction responds to sugar-fortified orange juice, but once confusion and coma supervene, parenteral therapy is mandatory.

Glucagon for injection, U.S.P., is laudable therapy, boasting ease and safety of home administration by family members. The dose is 1 mg of Glucagon dissolved in 1 ml of the accompanying diluting solution, injected literally anywhere—subcutaneously, intramuscularly, or intrave-

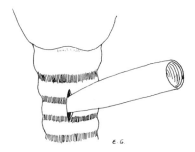

Fig. 12–5. In emergency tracheotomy, maintain the airway with the hollow
   barrel of a ballpoint pen.

nously—using the patient's own insulin syringe. Within a few minutes,
the patient regains consciousness, and oral feedings are resumed. All
my insulin-dependent diabetic patients keep a package of Glucagon at
home for possible emergency use.

Arterial occlusion of the lower extremity is a surgical emergency. The
telephone rings insistently at 2 A.M.; Mr. Jones reports the sudden onset
of excruciating pain associated with coldness and pallor of one foot. Do
not, repeat do not, instruct Mr. Jones to elevate his foot, apply heat, and
call you in the morning. Your patient has described the symptoms and
physical findings of sudden arterial occlusion of the lower extremity,
and prompt surgical intervention is mandatory. Get out of your nice
warm bed and go see Mr. Jones. You may save his leg.

Thermal burns are common household injuries, often prompting telephone calls to your office. Immediate immersion in cold water arrests
thermal injury and anesthetizes damaged nerve endings. Don't use ice;
frostbite can result. Instruct your office nurse to tell the patient to
immerse the burn in cold water for 15 minutes before reporting to your
office for examination, and to specifically discourage the application of
greasy ointments which will have to be removed a few minutes later
in the office.

High fevers in infants abound in winter, attributed to everything
from teething to tonsillitis. Mothers confuse fever with the illness itself,
but you wouldn't make that mistake. Fever is a symptom. Diagnose and
treat the cause; then instruct the mother to treat the fever with aspirin
and possibly judicious sponging with tepid water as necessary until the
acute illness subsides.

"Doctor, Johnny's temperature is 103°. Can I give him an alcohol
bath?" No! Alcohol sponging of infants has been reported to cause
hypoglycemia with hypothermia, extensor rigidity, and convulsions.

Sponging is the practical application of refrigeration—a lowering of skin temperature as water evaporates. Ice cold water and alcohol are unnecessary and dangerous; instruct the mother to use water about room temperature and allow time for evaporation. That's what does the cooling.

Infant poisoning may involve any chemical in the home—from perfume to pesticide. Mercifully, most children sample a drop and sensibly reject the poison, causing no more problem than a few more gray hairs for mother. Sometimes, a minimal amount of household poison is ingested, and in these cases, the universal antidote is recommended. Useful also in youngsters who have ingested strong acid or alkali when emesis or lavage is contraindicated, the universal antidote is prepared at follows:

Two parts activated charcoal
One part magnesium oxide
One part tannic acid
Add to 1 to 2 oz of water

A foreign body causing airway obstruction in a child is often better removed by gravity than by forceps. Send the parents out of the room. Then hold the child upside down, tapping his head on the examination table or on a cushion placed on the floor. The obstructing foreign body is usually easily dislodged.

References and Suggestions for Further Reading

1. Bennett J C, Demos G D: Drug Abuse and What We Can Do About It. Springfield, Ill, Thomas, 1971.
2. Birch C A: Emergencies in Medical Practice. Baltimore, Williams & Wilkins, 1971.
3. Brooks S H, Nahum A M, Siegel A W: Causes of injury in motor vehicle accidents. Surg Gynecol Obstet 131:185–197, 1970.
4. Dreisbach R H: Handbook of Poisoning: Diagnosis and Treatment. Los Altos, Calif, Lange, 1969.
5. Eckert C: Emergency-Room Care. Boston, Little, Brown, 1967.
6. Feingold B F, Benjamini E, Michaeli D: The allergic responses to insect bites. Annu Rev Entomol 13:137–158, 1968.
7. Flint T J, Cain H D: Emergency Treatment and Management, 4th ed. Philadelphia, Saunders, 1970.
8. Gottschalk L A: Psychoactive drug use. Arch Gen Psychiatry 25:395–397, 1971.
9. Halikas J A, Goodwin D W, Guze S B: Marihuana effects. JAMA 217:692–694, 1971.
10. Hollister L E: Chemical Psychoses: LSD and Related Drugs. Springfield, Ill, Thomas, 1968.

11. Imperi L L, Kleber H D, Davie J S: Use of hallucinogenic drugs on campus. JAMA 204:1021–1024, 1968.

12. Kolansky H: Effects of marihuana on adolescents and young adults. JAMA 216:-486–492, 1971.

13. Louria D B: Medical complications of pleasure-giving drugs. Arch Int Med 123:-82–87, 1969.

14. Lund I, Lind B: Aspects of resuscitation. Proceedings of the Second International Symposium on Emergency Resuscitation, Oslo, Norway, 1967. Acta Anaesthesiol Scand, Suppl 29, 1968.

15. Rose N J, Schnurrenberger P R, Martin R J: Rabies prophylaxis. Arch Environ Health 23:57–60, 1971.

16. Spitzer S, Oaks W W, Moyer J J: Emergency Medical Management. New York, Grune & Stratton, 1971.

17. Stahnke H L: The Treatment of Venomous Bites and Stings. Tempe, Ariz, Arizona State University Bureau of Publications, 1966.

18. Steele R W, Tanaka P T, Lara R P, Bass J W: Evaluation of sponging and/or oral antipyretic therapy to reduce fever. J Pediatr 77:824–829, 1970.

19. String T, Robinson A J, Blaisdell F W: Massive trauma. Arch Surg 102:406–411, 1971.

13

The Laboratory Is Your Friend

It is by testing that we discern fine gold.

Leonardo da Vinci

The laboratory is a fickle mistress, petulantly slow, confounding your most righteous intentions, but rising to support you in troubled times. Curse her caprice and condemn her follies, but don't try to get along without her. When the roll is called, the laboratory is your friend.

HEMATOLOGY

Drawing a blood sample is the first step in hematology, and it's a cumbersome one when your patient's veins lie submerged beneath subcutaneous fat. Don't look for the vein; feel for it. Take your time searching; the longer the tourniquet is in place, the more distended the veins become. Liberal swabbing with alcohol followed by a brisk slap helps bring shy veins to the surface.

Here's a tip for visualizing hidden veins: Don your red x-ray lenses. The veins stand out like expressways on a roadmap.

Found the vein? Then pierce the skin quickly, lateral to the vein, and stop. Withdraw the plunger slightly to create a vacuum; then pierce the vein. As the vein wall is punctured, you will feel a barely discernible pop and see the sudden rush of blood into your syringe.

Capillary blood can be used in determining the hemoglobin, hematocrit, white blood cell, red blood cell, reticulocyte, and platelet values—obviating the need for venipuncture. For obscure reasons, patients prefer a finger-stick. I routinely draw blood from the ring finger, less likely than the others to be used later that day. Prick the lateral finger pad and spare the complex nerve endings in the finger tip. Wash with alcohol, then dry thoroughly lest your results reflect artificial dilution. Grasp the finger firmly and stab with your lancet in a single bold stroke. If you prick lightly, you will probably have to repeat the procedure. Wipe away the first drop of blood and use the following drops for your determinations; avoid squeezing tissue fluid into the sample, since this may cause hemodilution.

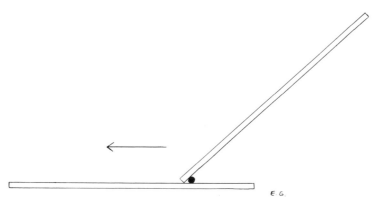

Fig. 13–1. To make a blood smear, spread the drop briskly but smoothly.

The **hemoglobin determination** tells the grams of hemoglobin per 100 ml of whole blood. The normal range is 12 to 18 gm, varying with the age, sex, and nutritional status of the patient. A low hemoglobin value is a symptom, not a diagnosis; it occurs with iron deficiency, blood dyscrasia, hemorrhage, and a host of other ills. An elevated hemoglobin value is of less clinical significance, although it is found in emphysema, dehydration, diarrhea, congestive heart failure, and of course, true polycythemia—rare as a robin in January.

The **hematocrit** measures the volume of red blood cells, packed by centrifugation, as a percentage of the volume of whole blood. The normal range is from 35 to 55 percent, also varying with age and sex. The office laboratory usually employs a microhematocrit determination, a more precise measurement of increases and decreases in the red blood cells than either the hemoglobin determination or the red blood cell count.

The microhematocrit capillary tubes may be filled with venous or capillary blood; fresh venous blood permits the most accurate determinations. Beware of prolonged centrifugation: it may lead to hemolysis and erroneously low values. And remember to seal the end of the tube to prevent leakage, lest your healthy patient appear to have a profound anemia.

The "anemia of pregnancy" is often diagnosed on the basis of a hematocrit of 32 percent during the fourth or fifth month of pregnancy. Of course, Mrs. America-in-waiting probably also has ankle edema, swollen fingers, and puffy eyes. Her "anemia" may well be hemodilution, and iron tablets will produce little physiologic change except constipation.

The **blood smear** is a useful office procedure. A single drop of blood from finger-tip puncture or from the venipuncture needle is deposited at one end of a clean glass slide. A second slide is moved at a 30° angle to engage the drop (Fig. 13–1), then moved swiftly back to produce a smooth film with an elliptical border and covering more than one-half of the glass slide (Fig. 13–2).

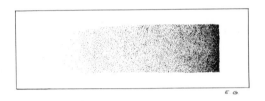

Fig. 13–2. A well-spread blood smear.

Dry the smear thoroughly before staining, but avoid undue delay which results in poor staining of white blood cells. In a hurry to stain? Can't wait for air-drying? Then dip the smear in 100 percent methanol and stain immediately.

"Lymphocytosis" is a frequent diagnostic coup of the neophyte technician. In fact, the overstained differential blood smear is the most common cause of lymphocytosis.

Two more tips: (1) Rouleau stacking of the red blood cells like poker chips suggests multiple myeloma; (2) a high eosinophil count, up to 80 percent, may be the tip-off to trichinosis.

The **bleeding time** is accurately determined after drawing capillary blood by lancet finger-tip puncture. Simply wipe the wound with a clean gauze pad every 30 seconds until bleeding ceases. The time elapsed is the bleeding time; normal value is 3 to 5 minutes.

The **coagulation time** is just as easy to determine. Fill a capillary tube with finger-tip or venous blood and use a Kelly clamp to break small pieces from the end at 1-minute intervals (Fig. 13–3). Continue until coagulation is demonstrated by a thick fibrin clot; usually 3 to 5 minutes is needed.

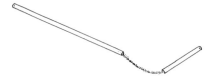

Fig. 13–3. To determine coagulation time, look for the fibrin clot.

The **partial thromboplastin time** has become a useful screening test for clotting abnormalities. It reflects a deficiency of the intrinsic pathway factors, circulating anticoagulants, or fibrinogen breakdown products, but not of factor VII or platelets. The normal partial thromboplastin time is 35 to 50 seconds; values less than 35 seconds, reflecting enhanced coagulability, are of questionable clinical significance.

URINE ANALYSIS

The urine specimen should be submitted in a clean, transparent container, although I have received samples in old peanut-butter jars, cider jugs, and even one in a foil-wrapped jar with a daffodil sticking in it. Your snap-top plastic medicine vials make excellent urine specimen containers; when the patient submits his specimen from home, give him a plastic vial to use next time.

It's often important to obtain a urine specimen from an infant. Don't try to wring out wet lint-filled diapers. Use Scotch Brand Magic Mending Tape to affix a plastic sandwich bag (Baggie) over the child's external genitalia. The next flood fills the bag, affording you an adequate specimen. Want to be really fancy? Then stock the commercially prepared infant urine specimen collectors—expensive baggies with adhesive tape in place.

Cloudy urine may cloud the diagnosis, making a specimen appear much more abnormal than it is. Dissolve those precipitated crystals and the specimen may be sparkling clear. Urates (Fig. 13–4) precipitate in acid urine and dissolve when alkali is added; thus cloudy urine with an acid pH will often clear when 10% potassium hydroxide is added.

Cloudy urine with an alkaline pH reflects precipitated phosphates

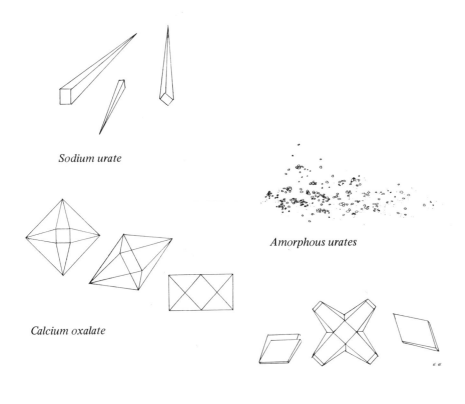

Sodium urate

Amorphous urates

Calcium oxalate

Uric acid crystals

Fig. 13–4. Crystals found in acid urine.

(Fig. 13–5). These dissolve when hydrochloric acid or white vinegar is added.

Bili-Labstix have taken the sorcery out of urine analysis. A single dip-stick reveals pH, protein, glucose, ketones, bilirubin, and blood. The pH, the clue to the composition of urinary crystals, achieves clinical significance in determining solubility of calculus-forming urates and cystine. Unexpected proteinuria may indicate nephrosis, chronic glomerulonephritis, diabetic nephropathy, or any acute febrile illness.

The finding of **glycosuria** may reflect diabetes or simply a high carbohydrate meal eaten an hour before. Many an unexpectedly glycosuric patient has recently breakfasted on toast with honey. If a repeat test also indicates glycosuria or if clinical findings suggest diabetes, the patient

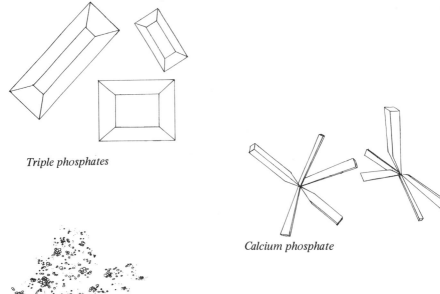

Triple phosphates

Calcium phosphate

Amorphous phosphates

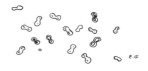

Calcium carbonate

Fig. 13–5. Crystals found in alkaline urine.

should have a blood glucose test to differentiate true diabetes from renal glycosuria.

Think you can check out your laboratory by submitting a urine sample laced with table sugar? Forget it! Bili-Labstix and other standard laboratory tests detect glucose, not sucrose.

Ketonuria may indicate acidosis or toxemia, but is often found in healthy children on routine physical examination, and in these cases is of no clinical significance. Use your head and relate the urinary ketone findings to the patient: No other clinical abnormalities, no significance.

Urinary bilirubin parallels hyperbilirubinemia, and blood should be drawn for confirmation. The most common causes are infectious hepatitis and obstructive jaundice.

Blood in the urine is a real danger sign. Although acute cystitis may cause transient hematuria, the repeated microscopic detection of red blood cells in the urine should prompt thorough urologic investigation. Painless hematuria is the most common finding in cancer of the urinary tract.

The **urinary salicylate test** can yield valuable data in seconds, while the harried night laboratory technician is explaining why she can't run your test for at least 2 hours. To 5 ml of heated urine, add 1 ml of 10% ferric chloride solution and shake gently. A purple color indicates that one of the following compounds is present: acetylsalicylic acid, phenol derivatives, sodium, phenyl, or methyl salicylate. One caution: The ferric chloride test is qualitative, not quantitative.

Red urine is passed by a child and tests negative for blood on Bili-Labstix. What can it be? Here's your chance for a shrewd diagnostic coup. Ask the mother, "Did Johnny have beets for dinner?" If he did, the red color is beet pigment in the urine, of no clinical significance.

Remember the country doctor's test for **bile in the urine** when you're called to the hippie commune and you think your patient may have hepatitis. Shake the urine in a closed, transparent container. White foam is normal; yellow foam indicates that bile is present.

BLOOD CHEMISTRY

The office laboratory, although threatened by the computers that beget multiple determinations from a single small sample, still boasts low initial cost and on-the-spot convenience. I use the Biodynamics Unitest system; Flint Diagnostics and Ames manufacture equally reliable systems. While the patient or his specimen is still on the way to the magic autoanalyzer at the county laboratory, your office lab has the results in hand.

Normal values for blood components vary with the procedure used. Your own report form should contain the range of normals for your system, and the county laboratory should be encouraged to do the same.

A centrifuge is required to spin down samples for determination of serum values. Be sure to buy one that can be used for both blood and urine samples. The heavy centrifuge is usually stationary by virtue of its bulk, but the small office centrifuge may dance a wild flamenco on the counter even though carefully balanced. Restrain your centrifuge's dancing by mounting it on foam rubber to absorb vibration.

Fasting blood specimens are recommended for most chemical determinations. By the time you return from the hospital at 10 A.M., your breakfast-less patient is weak in the knees, and following venipuncture, hypoglycemic syncope becomes a real possibility, particularly if the patient is scheduled for a physical examination along with his blood tests. We serve "breakfast at doctor's." The office routinely stocks orange juice, doughnuts, and hot coffee—a welcome collation for the patient anticipating a full physical examination.

The **fasting blood sugar** determination, the routine screening test for diabetes mellitus, is reliable for following the progress of the disease, but not for diagnosing it. For diagnosis, the *sine qua non* is the glucose tolerance test. Pretty sure of your diagnosis? Don't feel the full glucose tolerance test is needed? Then do the 2-hour postprandial blood sugar test, the most important determination in the 3-hour glucose tolerance test. That single glucose determination, made on blood drawn 2 hours after a 100-gm glucose test meal, will detect the vast majority of diabetics.

What is the significance of a high **cholesterol** value in a healthy young woman? Check her thyroid. The hypercholesterolemia may be the tip-off to hypothyroidism.

The **blood urea nitrogen** value should be determined annually for all patients with suspected chronic urinary tract infection, stricture, chronic glomerulonephritis, or diabetic uropathy. A misleading BUN elevation may be caused by dehydration and is associated with similar rises in hematocrit, hemoglobin, uric acid, and blood sugar values.

The **serum bilirubin** determination compensates for the eye's inability to detect jaundice if the serum bilirubin level is less than 2.0 mg per 100 ml. The office bilirubin determination allows accurate assessment of hepatitis and obstructive jaundice.

The **serum glutamic oxaloacetic transaminase** (SGOT) determination is important in two conditions that won't wait 3 days for the county laboratory to return results to you: acute infectious hepatitis and suspected myocardial infarction. The SGOT value denotes acute liver damage in hepatitis. It can be as important as the electrocardiogram in the early diagnosis of suspected coronary artery occlusion.

Thyroid function tests include more than the determination of basal metabolism rate. Blood triiodothyronine (T_3) and thyroxine (T_4) values are usually elevated in hyperthyroidism and decreased in hypothyroidism. An abnormally high T_3 value is also found in the patient taking diphenylhydantoin, androgens, or salicylates. A falsely high T_4 value accompanies the use of oral contraceptives or estrogens and is noted in pregnancy. Can't remember all that? Then order the T_7—the product of the T_3 and T_4 values—a calculation that discounts the action of outside factors on the T_3 and T_4 values. Normal ranges for T_7 values vary with each laboratory performing the tests.

THROAT CULTURE

The throat culture for streptococcus is rapid, inexpensive, and easy to read—a vast improvement over the previous "clinician's best guess" method of diagnosing streptococcal infection. Disposable blood-agar plates cost about 40 cents each. Material from the throat can be smeared directly on the plate by means of a cotton-tipped applicator, and the results are read in 18 to 24 hours. A clear zone of beta hemolysis indicates the presence of streptococci.

An office incubator is a necessity. The cost is less than $100. Use the machine to incubate Trans-Grow GC cultures before they are transported to the laboratory; use its warm top for drying Pap slides and blood smears.

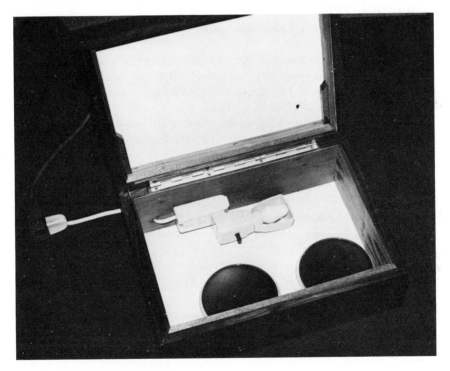

Fig. 13–6. The homemade incubator.

Throat cultures on weekends need present no problem. An inexpensive home incubator is easily constructed (Fig. 13–6). Drill some holes in the back of an ordinary cigar humidor and introduce an electric extension cord through one of them (the others are for ventilation). Plug in an ordinary nightlight. You may find your homemade incubator works better than your office model.

SPUTUM EXAMINATION

The sputum specimen may resist production, the patient emitting only a dry, barking cough. Give this patient a big glass of water and a double dose of one of your samples of an expectorant containing glyceryl guiacolate (but no codeine). Still no specimen? Patient a smoker? Let him have a smoke; the productive cough will probably begin.

A **gram-stained sputum smear** allows bacteriologic evaluation, perhaps revealing staphylococci in gram-positive clusters, streptococci in gram-positive chains, or pneumococci in gram-positive pairs.

Fungus infections may be detected by adding India ink to the smear, accentuating the capsule.

Blood-tinged sputum is common in acute bronchitis and should subside promptly upon recovery from the infectious process. Persistent hemoptysis may signal laryngeal or bronchogenic carcinoma and requires intensive investigation.

Cytologic examination of sputum is a valuable tool in cancer detection, provided an alveolar specimen containing pulmonary histiocytes is submitted. A sample consisting of a little nasal mucus and saliva won't do. Have the patient rinse his mouth with saline prior to coughing. Then produce an alveolar specimen by means of postural drainage, perhaps assisted by a warm saline aerosol spray. The specimen should be expectorated directly into a 95% ethyl alcohol–ether solution and sent to the laboratory.

EXAMINATION OF FECES

Occult blood in the feces is detected with a Hematest tablet. The tablet placed in the center of a fecal smear on filter paper and 2 drops of water are placed on the tablet. As the water runs onto the filter paper, a blue color indicates the presence of occult blood. The test is quite sensitive, and a falsely positive reaction may result if the patient has recently eaten rare meat. If you're in doubt, repeat the test after 3 days during which the patient has eaten no meat.

The Hematest tablet can also be used to detect hidden blood in other body fluids, including urine, sputum, and gastric contents.

Pinworms lurk in the dark recesses of the rectum, sallying forth at night to cause intense anal itching but hiding safe and warm within the lower bowel during the day. Try as she may, with flashlight in hand, the suspicious mother cannot find the thread-like worms. So she brings her squirming, itching offspring to you.

The NIH swab, an imposing eponym for a simple clinical device, uses cellophane tape to pick up pinworm ova from the anal area, allowing microscopic identification. I use Scotch Brand Magic Mending Tape; I'm sure it works as well as the National Institute of Health brand. Press the tape, sticky side down, against the anus. Then affix the tape, still sticky side down, to a glass slide and invert the slide, viewing through the glass rather than through the tape. If present, the pinworm ova are readily visible.

PREGNANCY TEST

A screening test for pregnancy can answer a lot of questions. Of the many tests available, most utilizing similar biochemical reactions, I now use the Pregnosticon slide test. When the directions are carefully followed and the urine sufficiently concentrated, the results are reliable, but not foolproof.

Wait 3 weeks after the missed menstrual period. A falsely negative reaction may result from hasty testing, before sufficient time has elapsed to allow development of detectable gonadotropins in the urine.

A falsely positive reaction may occur in a girl taking birth control pills sporadically or a menopausal woman who has infrequent menstrual periods and a high urinary gonadotropin level.

Legal implications sometimes accompany the possibly pregnant patient. Is she 14 years old? Is there a divorce in the offing? Has her husband been in Vietnam for the past 12 months? Then be sure the specimen submitted belongs to the patient; don't accept a sample brought from home. And have your results confirmed by the county laboratory.

THAT SPECIMEN BELONGS TO A PATIENT

Laboratory errors are distressingly common. Specimens get hot, cold, hemolyzed, contaminated, mislabeled, spilled, or lost. Most erroneous laboratory reports are caused by personal error on the part of technicians. Your clinical judgment is superior to any laboratory test ever devised, and when the lab report belies your clinical judgment, trust your eyes and ears; then repeat the laboratory test.

Help the lab by telling them what you have in mind. What is your tentative diagnosis? What are you looking for? Where did the specimen come from? How old is the patient? Any antibiotics used recently? What are you really looking for? The pathologist likes to think he is "the doctor's doctor;" give him a little history to work with.

Report test results to the patient. After all, he's the one who paid for them and who hopes they will help him get well. No patient should be told, "I'll call you only if the lab report indicates an abnormality." That patient never *really* knows if you saw the test report.

Preprinted cards facilitate reporting of routine tests of all types (Fig. 13–7). Is the situation urgent or delicate? Then telephone the patient personally. Following the conversation, on the back of the laboratory slip or in your clinical record, summarize the conversation, including the date and time.

Robert B. Taylor, M.D.
66 Forest Glen Road
New Paltz, New York 12561

Telephone:
255-5450

Date: ....

This is a report of the results of your recent test(s):

NAME:

TEST(S):

RESULTS:

Very truly yours,
Dr. Taylor

Fig. 13–7. Laboratory report card.

Plan a repeat test? Then inform the patient, make sure he has the proper requisition, put a reminder card in your monthly tickler file, and record your recommendation in the patient's clinical record.

References and Suggestions for Further Reading

1.   Adams J T, Clermont G H, Schwartz S I: Acute cholecystitis and serum transaminase activity. Arch Surg 101:366–369, 1970.

2.   Benson E S, Strandjord P E: Multiple Laboratory Screening. New York, Academic Press, 1969.

3.   Breese B B, Disney F A: The accuracy of diagnosis of beta streptococcal infections on clinical grounds. J Pediatr 44:670–673, 1954.

4. Davidsohn I, Henry J B: Clinical Diagnosis by Laboratory Methods. Philadelphia, Saunders, 1969.

5. Goodale R H, Widmann F K: Clinical Interpretation of Laboratory Tests, 6th ed. Philadelphia, Davis, 1969.

6. Kelley T G: Automation revolution in laboratory medicine. Mod Med 37:44–52, 1969.

7. Levinson S A, MacFate R P: Clinical Laboratory Diagnosis, 7th ed. Philadelphia, Lea & Febiger, 1969.

8. Macdougal L G: Simple test for detection of iron in stools. J Pediatr 76:764–765, 1970.

9. Natelson S: Techniques of Clinical Chemistry. Springfield, Ill, Thomas, 1971.

10. Schoen I, Thomas G D, Lange S: Quality of performance in physicians' office laboratories. Am J Clin Pathol 55:163–170, 1971.

11. Starr P: Hypercholesterolemia in school children: Preliminary report. Am J Clin Pathol 56:515–522, 1971.

12. Wallach J: Interpretation of Diagnostic Tests. Boston, Little, Brown, 1970.

14

Prevention Is
Better Than Treatment

And lo! the starry folds reveal
  The blazoned truth we hold so dear:
To guard is better than to heal—
  The shield is nobler than the spear!

Oliver Wendell Holmes
(1809–1894)

The doctor toils diligently to put himself out of business, striving for a Utopia where all diseases are conquered and accidents prevented. Thousands of medical students tacitly assume failure of the quest, confident in the proliferation of bacteria, the deterioration of aging organs, and the inevitability of accidents.

But while the tireless family physician plods through his day, bright young scientists are unlocking the mysteries of infections, cancer, and heart disease—trying to develop effective vaccines, diets, and prophylaxis against disease. As each year passes, the clinician will spend less time treating sick patients and more hours will be devoted to disease prevention.

THE ROUTINE PHYSICAL EXAMINATION

The routine physical examination is the backbone of preventive medicine. You can't improve your patient's health until you get him in the office. Once there, update his medical history, check his blood pressure and weight, remove his clothes and perform a thorough physical examination. Then alert him to the early signs of illness—nagging heartburn, morning cough, increasing weight, and rising blood sugar level. Discuss his work, diet, and habits; prescribe any modification necessary to improve health.

Exercise judgment and restraint. The patient with a fasting blood sugar value of 115 mg per 100 ml needs weight reduction, not a rigid diabetic exchange diet. A serum cholesterol value of 270 mg per 100 ml calls for restriction of fried eggs, ice cream, and those cheese snacks at night; a prescription for Atromid-S is not indicated. Few middle-aged housewives have the figure of Raquel Welch, but modest weight reduction is often in order. Sensible preventive advice leads to confident compliance, but dogmatic repressive schedules usually end in the wastebasket of frustration.

Physical examinations in children are usually prompted by the mother's need to have a form completed for school or camp. Here's your chance to do a good job. Check the height-weight percentiles, discuss the youngster's eating habits, inquire about his school performance, give him a thorough physical examination, and bring his immunizations up-to-date.

Here's a time-saving tip in performing the school or camp physical exam: When the mother telephones for an appointment, your aide should instruct her to fill in "her part" of the form, including the child's past medical history and immunizations. Also instruct the mother to please, please bring in the child's urine specimen; few youngsters can void on command and precious office minutes are wasted while the youngster dawdles, runs water in the lavatory, and awaits the urge to urinate.

Routine physical examinations on sick children should be discouraged. "While Johnny's here with his fever and earache, doctor, would you fill out this form?" Usually Johnny's acute illness has justified squeezing him into an already bulging schedule. Explain to his mother that the thorough physical examination involves hearing tests, vision tests, and effort on Johnny's part. "He's just too sick today; let's schedule Johnny's examination for another time when he is feeling better."

The use of an oral contraceptive mandates an annual examination.

Don't skimp by performing a Pap test and confidently pronouncing the patient fit for another year. Allot the time, do a thorough examination, and then write an oral contraceptive prescription that will run out in 1 year, remembering that the calendar year has 13 lunar months, not 12.

A tuberculin skin test should be performed at intervals, depending upon household and community likelihood of exposure. With the passing years, fewer and fewer adults show positive tuberculin reactions, and the recent conversion of a previously negative reacter warrants thorough testing and x-ray examination of all household members. Apply the Tine Test firmly, but don't draw blood. Then use a felt-tipped or ballpoint pen to draw a ring around the test site so you can find it 2 or 3 days later. Capable mothers can be relied upon to return their charges if a positive reaction is noted, but the parent with marginal reliability should be scheduled for a revisit to read the Tine Test.

Robert B. Taylor, M.D.   Telephone:
66 Forest Glen Road   255-5450
New Paltz, N. Y. 12561

Name: Anne Marie Smith

Yes, it's that time already!
Don't Forget to call for an appointment.

   X   Annual Physical Examination

........Chest X-ray

........Electrocardiogram

........Regular Check-Up

........Flu Shot

........Poison Ivy Shot

   X   Rubella Vaccine

Fig. 14–1. Reminder card.

A tickler file enables your secretary to jog your patient's lagging memory. Some physicians schedule routine physical examinations near the patient's birthday, but this method seems cumbersome. A reminder card (Fig. 14-1) effectively alerts the forgetful patient that routine physical examination time is near. Fill in the reminder card while the patient is still in the office, file the card by month of the year, and 3, 6, or 12 months from now, check the card (making sure Mrs. Jones wasn't in the office yesterday), and out it goes in the mail.

TEACH YOUR PATIENTS GOOD HEALTH HABITS

Good health habits help prevent illness. How many of your daily consultations concern ulcer patients who swill coffee by the pint, emphysematous chain smokers, construction workers who have never mastered the art of lifting, and obese gourmands? It is better to be healthy and rich than sick and poor.

Backache is better prevented than treated. Patient instruction in cautious habits of lifting, bending, sitting, and standing can minimize recurrences of low back strain. Here's a list of tips for your patients with low back strain. Copy on your letterhead, duplicate, and let your patients study these rules while nestled under the diathermy machine:

RULES TO HELP PREVENT BACKACHE

1. Use your strong leg muscles to lift. Never bend from the waist.
2. Avoid standing for long periods of time.
3. When lifting, face the object, get your balance, think about your back, and bend your knees.
4. Never move furniture, push a stalled car, or attempt to lift very heavy objects alone.
5. When sitting, try to bend your knees so they are higher than your hips. Use a footstool whenever possible.
6. Avoid deep chairs and soft couches. Your back prefers firm chairs and mattresses.
7. Wear only low-heeled, firm walking shoes. Women should avoid high heels.
8. Never hold an object at arm's length. It exerts a tremendous strain on the low back.
9. Rest one foot on a box or "bar rail," locking the hips and resting the back muscles when standing.
10. Exercise regularly to maintain youthful muscle tone.

Heart disease smites men in the prime of life. In *Pathology for the Surgeon*, William Boyd wrote: "Of all the ailments which may blow out life's little candle, heart disease is the chief." The coronary artery occlusion shocks 50-year-old company vice president William Brown and his family, but comes as no surprise to his physician, who has for years admonished Bill to work fewer hours, dine less extravagantly, cut down his smoking, and exercise more often. Direct your patients' attention to these good health habits and you will care for less devastating myocardial infarctions.

Salt enhances the flavor of food, is an essential body compound, increases the intravascular fluid volume, contributes to hypertension, and aggravates congestive heart failure. Few elderly patients can afford the luxury of excessive salt consumption. Salt-free foods are expensive and rarely necessary, but neither should sodium chloride be added at the table. Co-Salt contains potassium chloride and ammonium chloride, and can safely be recommended for any salt-restricted patient unless he suffers from coexistent oliguria or severe kidney disease.

Obesity is a bad habit, usually the just desserts of compulsive consumption of excessive quantities of rich food. Help your patient break the obesity habit by directing his chocolate-cake craving to a celery compulsion. Ice water has considerably fewer calories than alcoholic beverages. Recent studies have related adult obesity to infant overfeeding—excessive fat cells formed during the first few months of life. Start early to combat overfeeding by encouraging dietary restrictions and skim milk feedings for chubby infants.

Diaper rash begins with poor laundry habits. To get her baby's diapers snowy white, Mrs. Clean uses the strongest detergent she can find —usually Tide, All, or Cold Power. The diapers are beautifully white, but the baby's bottom is red, as urine dissolves residual soap particles to attack the protective fatty layers of his skin. Specifically recommend Ivory Snow or Fels Naptha; tell Mrs. Clean to use a little less soap than she thinks she should and to run the diapers through a second rinse to remove residual soap particles.

Infant tooth decay has been traced to indolent bottle-sucking. The milk-encrusted nipple forms an excellent culture medium for bacteria. Instruct the mother to feed the baby, empty the bottle, then carefully scrub bottle and nipple and put them away.

DISEASE PREVENTION

Disease transmission may begin in your office if a well baby is allowed to play with a child who has a strep throat. Here's where your aides must use their heads. Rush sick patients through the waiting room; bring patients known or suspected to have contagious diseases in by the back door. Use your consultation room or the nurses' station as a waiting room for such patients until an examination room is vacant.

Otitis media can sometimes be prevented by conscientious administration of decongestants and nosedrops to the ear-infection-prone patient with a common cold. If eustachian tube patency is maintained, infection is often thwarted. Aerotitis media, resulting from an air pressure differential across the eardrum as the airplane descends, can often be prevented if the traveler takes a decongestant, uses a nasal spray, and swallows repeatedly during descent. Before the days of pressurized aircraft, the stewardess distributed candy and gum; now martinis are handed round as a concession to commercialism and improved, but not perfected, pressurization.

Hexachlorophene soaps, darlings of Madison Avenue in the 1960s, are suffering the end of the honeymoon with doctors and the Food and Drug Administration. Maybe it's true that "too much bathing weakens a man." Excessive use of hexachlorophene soap has resulted in sensitization and dry skin. As in other organs, destruction of the bacterial flora of the skin may lead to monilial infection. Systemic absorption has been linked to brain damage. I specifically advise new mothers to avoid hexachlorophene soap (in spite of specious advertising) in favor of a good old-fashioned mild baby soap, such as Johnson's.

Infectious hepatitis prevention causes more annoyance than treatment of the disease itself. Why does each new hepatitis patient always seems to have attended a large festive gathering two nights before. Here's your critierion for gamma-globulin administration: Give gamma globulin to every person who shared food with your patient during the preceding week, including all household contacts. Classmates, casual acquaintances, and friends of household contacts require no prophylactic therapy. Your patient spent the night at the party, sharing food, drink, and embraces with the assembled multitude? Then you had better inject each of them with gamma globulin in a dose of 0.01 ml per pound of body weight. I usually give a little extra by rounding up to the next even half milliliter.

Diabetes mellitus may not be preventable but its onset can often be delayed. Some folks simply eat themselves into diabetes. The dormant metabolic defeat, passed from generation to generation, is activated by excessive carbohydrate consumption and gross obesity. Have a prediabetic patient? Borderline blood sugar level? Strong family history? Then insist that he maintain his ideal weight and reduce his carbohydrate consumption to the minimum. This will delay the day he crosses the obscure line into overt diabetes.

Insect bites plague adults and children during summer months, ravenous insects often seeking out the fair-skinned blond. Advise the bite-prone patient not to lure insects to herself with flowered print dresses and scented soaps. Insect repellents are of short-term value. Some physicians recommend vitamin B_2 (riboflavin) as an insect repellent;

apparently the vitamin changes the chemical composition of sweat in a manner inimical to insects but undetectable to humans. Give it a try: A 5-mg riboflavin tablet taken two or three times daily.

Poison ivy dermatitis is preventable. Avoidance of the plant is laudable but often difficult. One or two applications of an inexpensive herbicide will eradicate nearby growths of poison ivy; but then in comes the dog with the ivy oleoresin carried invisibly on his fur. The patient's resistance to poison ivy can be enhanced by hyposensitization using Ivyol in a first-year series of four 0.5 ml injections weekly, followed by a single 0.5 ml booster annually in the spring. Your patient already has poison ivy? Then treat him with full-dosage corticosteroids, withholding Ivyol until the skin is clear. Ivyol hyposensitization is less than 100 percent effective, and the patient should continue careful habits of avoidance and thorough scrubbing of all exposed areas following a romp in the woods.

Vitamin C has been prescribed as poison ivy prophylaxis—another of the mystical powers attributed to this simple chemical compound. In my own limited and statistically insignificant series, the subjective patient response has been excellent to a dose of 500 to 750 mg of ascorbic acid daily.

Influenza vaccine seems more effective than poison ivy shots. I recommend flu vaccine for all elderly patients and any adult whose severe, prolonged febrile illness would cause medical or economic problems. That includes practically everybody, doesn't it? The well-purified Fluogen vaccine is administered in 0.5 ml doses, the first injection in September followed by a booster dose approximately 2 to 3 months later. My high-risk patients receive two injections annually: The September dose protects for about 4 months; the second dose around the Christmas holidays affords protection until the tulips bloom and prevents the often-noted flu outbreak in February and March.

Cold shots lack the respectability of flu vaccine; they are infrequently indicated and are effective only in a limited number of highly suggestible people. Your patient with eight or ten common colds annually in spite of barely sublethal doses of vitamin C may respond to "cold shots." Cold vaccines are manufactured by a number of pharmaceutical companies, and there is no clearly superior preparation. Several supposedly ineffective vaccines, under FDA pressure, have been discontinued. Dosage schedules vary, and the manufacturer's recommendation should be followed.

ACCIDENT PREVENTION

Every child knows that prevention is not only better than cure, but also cheaper.

Henry E. Sigerist
Atlantic Monthly
June 1939

The prevented accident is an ambulance that wasn't called, a hospital bed that remained cold, a disability that didn't occur, and an idle afternoon you can spend on the golf course.

Medication and driving may be a hazardous combination, as law-enforcement officials and the public have recently discovered. Your patient involved in an automobile accident, major or minor, may be asked, "Are you taking any drugs?" The officer doesn't really think your patient, a respectable but drowsy middle-aged housewife, is shooting heroin; he's asking about tranquilizers, "tonic pills," antihistamines, or another of the vast host of drugs which can produce sedation. If your patient's accident caused serious bodily injury and she insists she didn't know the medication could cause drowsiness, the doctor could be in trouble.

When you prescribe a potentially sedative medication for a patient who drives, specifically caution him against operating machinery when under its influence, most particularly after taking the first dose or two. Then note the warning on the patient's clinical record and label the prescription, "Do not operate machinery while taking this medication."

Think I'm being too cautious? Your patient would never bring litigation against his friendly family doctor? That's right, he probably wouldn't. But the other driver will, and your patient's insurance company might.

Seatbelts save lives. We all know that, but how about lap belts worn by pregnant women? In 1971, Crosby and Costiloe reported on 208 pregnant victims of severe accidents, 28 wearing seatbelts and 180 unrestrained. Seat belts halved the maternal death rate (7.8 percent without seatbelts died compared with 3.6 percent with seatbelts), but caused a slight increase in the fetal loss rate (14.4 percent fetal loss in victims without seatbelts compared with 16.7 percent in those with seatbelts). More significant, however, were the findings that in severe collisions 33 percent of women ejected from the car died compared with 5 percent of women not ejected. The fetal death rate was 47 percent with ejection and 11 percent without, paralleling the maternal loss. Encourage your pregnant patients to use their lap belts.

Should grandpa drive a car? Here's a real problem, requiring the diplomacy of an ambassador and the authority of a prime minister. Grandpa's good eye will get him past the eye test, and he thinks he can stay on the road in spite of his tremor. Look at his record—45 years of driving without a citation until that "going too slow" ticket last year. But you know and the family knows that grandpa shouldn't drive. I use this question: "If your grandchild ran out in front of your car, could you stop in time?" Usually grandpa sees the implication and retires his license, but he may be prepared to argue. That's when you must take charge. "I'm sorry, my friend, but I don't think you could stop in time to avoid a running child. I must insist you leave the driving to younger family members with sharper eyes and quicker reflexes."

Wrist and hand lacerations occur as Billy opens the storm door by pushing too hard on the glass panel, shattering the pane. Nasty lacerations indeed, and completely preventable. As you make your house calls, notice the screen-storm doors. An unprotected pane in a household with children is an accident waiting for a time to happen. Point out the danger and advise the parents to buy an inexpensive aluminum shield, easily affixed to the door.

PREVENTIVE MEDICINE FOR THE TRAVELER

When meditating over disease, I never think of finding a remedy for it, but, instead, a means of preventing it.

> *Louis Pasteur*
> *Address to the Fraternal Association of Former Students*
> *of the Ecole Centrale des Arts et Manufactures, Paris, May 15, 1884*

Thanks to pioneers like Pasteur (he developed the first cholera vaccine for chickens, remember?), Edward Jenner, John Enders, Jonas Salk, Albert Sabin, and thousands of other white-coated unsung heroes, we can roam the globe, armed with antibodies to repel hostile invading microorganisms.

In the eyes of public health authorities, **smallpox vaccination** has a double image. One faction emphasizes the danger of scattered postvaccinial complications and the other warns that this highly communicable disease has a mortality rate of up to 40 percent and is resistant to all available remedies. My foreign travelers continue to be vaccinated against smallpox, and when the airport public health service functionary inquires, "What countries did you visit during the past 2 weeks?"

my patients have the confidence of possessing a validated International Vaccination Certificate.

Of course, the yellow vaccination certificate isn't worth a nickel until validated by your area's public health office. Your patient can take the yellow card there in person, but why not mail the card directly from your office, enclosing a stamped envelope addressed to the patient's home? In a few days, his stamped certificate arrives in the mail.

Diptheria, tetanus, and poliomyelitis immunizations should be brought up-to-date before foreign travel. Unless he has recently been immunized, the tourist receives a single 0.5-ml intramuscular booster dose of adult tetanus-diptheria vaccine and a single booster dose of Sabin Trivalent Oral Polio vaccine.

Typhoid fever immunization is advised for travelers entering areas where sanitary conditions are less than ideal. The primary immunization against typhoid fever consists of two 0.5-ml doses of vaccine administered at least 4 weeks apart. The primary immunization probably need never be repeated; adequate recall is usually obtained with a single 0.5-ml dose intramuscularly or a 0.1-ml dose intradermally. The intradermal booster dose avoids most of the constitutional side effects of typhoid vaccine.

Typhus vaccine is suggested for travelers to certain areas of Africa, Central America, and South America, particularly those persons who intend to visit rural areas. The regimen is two 0.5-ml subcutaneous doses 4 weeks or more apart, followed by 0.5-ml booster doses at 6- to 12-month intervals if necessary.

Cholera vaccine is strongly recommended for visitors to Southeast Asia and certain areas of the Middle East. Like smallpox vaccine, the cholera immunization must be recorded and validated on the International Vaccination Certificate. The primary immunization against cholera consists of two subcutaneous doses, the first is 0.5 ml and the second, given four or more weeks later, is 1.0 ml. Booster doses of 0.5 ml may be administered at 6-month intervals.

Yellow fever vaccination is advisable for travelers in South and Central America and Africa, where the disease is endemic. Available only at Yellow Fever Centers listed with the World Health Organization, the yellow fever vaccination is recorded and validated on the International Certificate of Vaccination, including the identification stamp of the center. A single 0.5-ml dose of vaccine is valid for 10 years.

Plague vaccine may be advisable for travelers to Vietnam, Cambodia, Laos, and areas of Africa or Asia where plague is enzootic. Adults receive two intramuscular 0.5-ml doses 4 weeks or more apart followed by a third 0.2-ml dose 4 to 6 weeks later. Booster doses are given every

ROBERT B. TAYLOR, M.D.
66 FOREST GLEN ROAD
NEW PALTZ, NEW YORK 12561
—
TELEPHONE 914-255-5450

Date_____

Name: _____

Address: _____

_____

FOR FOREIGN TRAVEL: Please fill only those items
checked:

___   Lomotil tablets; dispense___tablets; take 2
tablets every 6 hours for diarrhea.

___   Bonine 25 mg; dispense___tablets; chew 1 tablet
every 12 hours for motion sickness.

___   Vioform-hydrocortisone cream: dispense 20 gm;
apply to skin rash 3 times a day.

___   Tetracycline 250 mg; dispense___capsules; take
1 capsule 4 times a day for infection.

___   Placidyl 500 mg; dispense___capsules; take 1
capsule at bedtime as needed for sleep.

___   Aralen 250 mg tablets for malaria suppression;
dispense___tablets; take 2 tablets on the same
day each week, beginning 2 weeks before and
continued 8 weeks after possible malaria
exposure.

Pharmacist:

Identify all medications on package label.
No refills.

Robert B. Taylor, M.D.
BNDD No. 1234567

Fig. 14–2. Prescription medication form for travelers.

6 to 12 months while the traveler remains in an area where the disease
is prevalent.

Gamma globulin as prophylaxis against infectious hepatitis may be
given to travelers journeying to any area where fecal contamination

threatens drinking water. Your patient may gulp bottled water all day and contract hepatitis rinsing his toothbrush. The dose is 0.01 ml of gamma globulin per pound of body weight, injected intramuscularly. The time of administration should be delayed until 1 or 2 days before departure.

The traveler's **first-aid kit** should contain, along with bandages and aspirin, prescription medication that may be needed in Rome or Tokyo. The traveler's prescription form (Fig. 14-2) is a handy check list that saves time for the doctor.

References and Suggestions for Further Reading

1. Anderson T: Smallpox immunization. Practitioner 195:281–283 1965.
2. Anderson W: Boyd's Pathology for the Surgeon, 9th ed. Philadelphia, Saunders, 1967.
3. Carter E T: Residency training in preventive medicine. Arch Eviron Health 23:-397–401, 1971.
4. Cassel J C, Heyden S, Bartel A: Incidence of coronary heart disease by ethnic group, social class, and sex. Arch Intern Med 128:901–906, 1971.
5. Crosby W M, Costiloe J P: Safety of lap-belt restraint for pregnant victims of automobile collisions. N Engl J Med 284:632–636, 1971.
6. Doto I L, Furcolow M L, MacInnis F E: Size of tuberculin reaction. Arch Environ Health 23:392–396, 1971.
7. Ferrer H P: Screening for Health: Theory and Practice. New York, Appleton, 1968.
8. Laurie W: Prevention of myocardial infarction. Med J Aust 1:361–363, 1971.
9. Mann G V: Obesity, the nutritional spook. Am J Public Health 61:1491–1498, 1971.
10. Nutrition Source Book, Chicago, National Dairy Council, 1970
11. Pineda A A, Sall S, Sedlis A, Stone M L: Impact of cytologic screening program on a gynecologic malignancy service. Med Digest 17:44–49, 1971.
12. Schuman L M: Approaches to primary prevention of disease. Public Health Rep 85:1–10, 1970.
13. Sharp C L E H, Keen H: Presymptomatic Detection and Early Diagnosis. Baltimore, Williams & Wilkins, 1968.
14. Sweeney F J: Symposium on what's new in infectious diseases: Prevention and immunization. Med Clin North Am 51:579–846, 1967.
15. Tuft L: Immunization against influenza and typhoid fever by intradermal method. Ann Allergy 29:23–29, 1971.
16. Vaccines: Which, when, for whom? Emergency Med 3:65–71, 1971.
17. Whitcomb N: Incidence of positive skin tests among medical students. Ann Allergy 29:67–70, 1971.
18. Wilson J M G, Junger G: Principles and Practice of Screening Disease. New York, Columbia University Press, 1968.

15

Your Patient Has a Family

Patients and their families will forgive you for wrong diagnoses, but will rarely forgive you for wrong prognoses; the older you grow in medicine, the more chary you get about offering ironclad prognoses, good or bad.

Albert R. Lamb
Journal of Chronic Diseases
16:441, 1963

Your patient is but a single star in his family constellation; he boasts a host of relatives, with solicitous concern for his health—whether motivated by love, guilt, or avarice.

THE FAMILY CONSTELLATION

Your patient's family participates in his illness, whether the participation involves losing time from work to care for a child with the flu, nagging to the extent that a spouse's gastric mucosa becomes hypersecretive, or patiently irrigating an elderly parent's indwelling catheter. Are five active children the cause of Mrs. Brown's tension headaches? Can you trust Mrs. Green to call back if her son's croup gets worse?

Who lives at home? Is your patient married? How many children does he have? Do they live at home? Are there elderly grandparents in the household? Has the family structure changed recently—a new baby, a visiting uncle, or an ulcerogenic mother-in-law?

What is your patient's role at home? Who wears the pants? Who does the cooking and dishes? Are major decisions dogmatically dictated or shared? Do the children communicate with their parents or walk the fine line between self-expression and hippiedom?

Concerned relatives can help or hinder the physician. Last month a worried wife scheduled her husband for a comprehensive physical examination: "Yes, doctor, I want Harry to have a thorough check-up, blood tests, chest x-ray, and electrocardiogram—everything." But that's not what she told Harry. On the fateful morning, Harry rushed in, having allotted a few minutes in his busy schedule for a quick blood pressure check. But we had scheduled a 90-minute examiniation. Could this crisis have been prevented? Yes. Here's the secret. Get the *patient* on the phone. Try to confirm all comprehensive physical examination appointments the day before, stressing the time allocated and speaking directly to the patient whenever possible.

Telephone calls from panicky relatives can disrupt your schedule needlessly. "Doctor, you've got to come quickly, my husband's coughing and pale and can't catch his breath." Sounds like a real emergency. Dashing out the door, black bag in hand, you shout apologies over your shoulder to the restless waiting room inhabitants. You speed to the patient's house, rush in, and are greeted with, "Doctor, my wife shouldn't have bothered you. I've had a little cold for a week and was planning to make an appointment." Your ulcer bleeds a little because you know that you would be back at your office and on schedule if only you had insisted upon talking to the patient.

Relatives color historical data—children reacting to mothers and husbands reacting to wives. Have you ever met Mr. Milkquetoast, whose wife tells you how he feels? How about the elderly couple who disagree on every historical detail, "No, Martin, you haven't been sick 9 days; I'm sure it's been 10." Allow the domineering relative to tell her story, then dismiss her to the waiting room "while the patient is examined." Once liberated, your patient can tell his tale without fear of interruption.

Relatives calling for information can shatter your schedule with endless, time-consuming questions. Multiply this nuisance by several relatives per patient and you might as well cancel office hours. When you find that calls for progress reports are coming from multiple family members, instruct the family to designate a spokesman to deal with the doctor. Then keep the spokesman up to date about the patient's progress and refer the calls from Aunt Minnie and Uncle George to him.

Relatives are everywhere. Of course, you wouldn't discuss your patient with the elevator operator, waitress, cab driver, deliveryman, or janitor, but a careless word to a colleague may be overheard by someone else, and that someone else is always your patient's second cousin. I have blanched at the elevator conversation of interns; "I had to dig an impaction out of that crocky old Mrs. White in 913 again last night." Or, "The emergency room sure dropped the ball on that kid with the appendix yesterday." Ten to one "the kid's" mother is standing behind that intern in the elevator. Use discretion, and keep your consultations private.

PROGNOSIS AND THE FAMILY

Hippocrates cautioned: "In acute diseases, it is not quite safe to prognosticate either death or recovery."

The intern, confidently calling upon his wealth of experience, assures the family, "Everything is going to be all right." After a few years in practice, he hedges a little: "Nothing will be spared, and unless complications develop, the patient should pull through." Twenty years and a half million patients later, he cautions: "We'll do everything we can. Let's hope and pray for the best."

Be optimistic if the case gives you half a chance. Don't dash the patient's hopes, however irrational. I know a patient who visited a large medical center for radiation therapy of a metastatic breast lesion. Happily, pain disappeared and x-ray appearance returned to normal. The patient was elated until the radiation therapist discharged her with, "Don't worry, you'll be back within a few years." Sure, he was right, and beneath her veil of fantasy, the patient knew the truth. But the doctor didn't have to *tell* her.

While the physician's guarded optimism may be therapeutic for the patient, someone in the family must understand the true facts. Here's where that family spokesman comes in. Call him in for a conference when the patient isn't present. Lay your cards on the table, show him x-rays if indicated, discuss 5-year survival rates, and communicate as clear a picture as possible. But when he tries to pin you down to what will happen next and how long the patient will live, avoid the dogmatic answer. Give general answers, generous life expectancy ranges, and avoid the embarrassment of having the patient outlive your prognosis or, what's worse, failing to fulfill your optimistic prophecies.

Predict death, and your ego has a vested interest in the patient's demise.

BAD NEWS AND THE FAMILY

Communicating bad news is the art of sincerity. You can't learn compassion, but a few guidelines can be followed.

Deal with the strongest family member. A midnight call to elderly Mrs. Johnson to tell her of her husband's death may be met with an ominous silence interrupted by the sickening thump of a fainting body striking the floor. Avoid the crisis by breaking the news first to son, Bill Johnson, the hardheaded middle-aged businessman, who can drive over to his mother's home and be with her when she is told the bad news.

The newborn infant with a birth defect is a family tragedy. The mother, convalescing from her labor and delivery, is in a labile emotional state and ill-prepared to receive bad news. Whether the defect is a correctable clubfoot or mongolism, if you suspect the news will throw the mother into a tailspin, find the husband. Tell him, painting as lucid a picture as possible. Then go together to face the mother. You'll be glad you called in her husband for support.

Allow the patient to hope. In the second century, Galen remarked: "Confidence and hope do more good than physic." However dismal the prognosis, however blunt you have been with the family spokesman, caution relatives to allow the patient his hopeful fantasies. The preterminal leukemia victim searching newspapers for the breakthrough that will save his life is, indeed, tragic, but the very act of hoping for a breakthrough in cancer cure has comforted many patients through their final months. The family should prepare for the worst, but help the patient hope for the best.

Should the family be summoned to the bedside? As with a tracheotomy in the child with croup, the time to do it is when you think about it. "Yes, it might be well for the family to come." That trip to the bedside, whether across town or across the country, is therapeutic for your patient and for the family members he will leave behind.

Many patients die on schedule, progressively deteriorating, following the textbook disease pattern, culminating in death following a few final hours of hypotension and labored respiration. In most cases, the family would prefer to be present. Instruct the hospital floor nurses to let you know when death is imminent. Telephone the family yourself. "It looks as though your father's time has come. He can't hold out much longer. I thought you would want to know." That call before death allows the family to prepare, marshal resources, and alert distant relatives. The final event will come as no surprise to this family.

Death brings guilt feelings to the surface—the imagined slight, the daughter who didn't write, the son who couldn't send money, the wife who "should have called the doctor earlier," the grandchild who "should have come home from college sooner." The doctor, like the parish priest, must remove the burden of guilt from the family's collective shoulders. Reassure the family that they (and you) have done all that could be done. "We all did our best. Nothing was spared. Certainly no family could have done more."

The death call, to confirm the sudden demise of a patient at home, comes to all doctors. You've cared for the Smith family for years. One morning Uncle Charlie, who doesn't believe in doctors, is found cold in bed. Without your signature on a death certificate, Uncle Charlie becomes a coroner's case with no end of legal problems. Make the call, confirming Uncle Charlie's departure. Carry a small vial of meprobamate or other mild tranquilizer to leave with the bereaved family. Reassure the survivors that they can call you if needed for support during the next few difficult days. (And you had better mean it; hysteria is as common as gladioli at funerals.) Charge for a death call? Never do it. For this call, you'll be paid in the next world.

References and Suggestions for Further Reading

1. Anthony E J, Benedek T: Parenthood: Its Psychology and Psychopathology. Boston, Little, Brown, 1970.
2. Barcai A: Family therapy in treatment of anorexia nervosa. Am J Psychiatry 128:-286–290, 1971
3. Cole D: Overcoming the Fear of Death. New York, Macmillan, 1970.
4. Crawford C O: Health and the Family: A Medical-Sociological Analysis. New York, Macmillan, 1971.
5. Field M: Patients Are People: A Medical-Social Approach to Prolonged Illness, 3rd ed. New York, Columbia University Press, 1967.
6. Lewis F C: Patients, Doctors and Families. Garden City, N Y, Doubleday, 1968.
7. McFadden C J: Medical Ethics, 6th ed. Philadelphia, Davis, 1967.
8. Paykel E S, Prusoff B A, Uhlenhuth E H: Sealing of life events. Arch Gen Psychiatry 25:340–347, 1971.
9. Rees W D, Lutkins S G: Mortality of bereavement. Br Med J 4:13–15, 1967.
10. Schoenberg B, Carr A C, Peretz D, Kutscher A H: Loss and Grief: Psychological Management in Medical Practice. New York, Columbia University Press, 1970.
11. Wingert W A: Influence of family organization on utilization of pediatric emergency service. Pediatrics 42:743–751, 1969.

16

Colleagues Are To Consult

There are probably as many "kindly old specialists" as there are "kindly old family physicians."

Robert H. Ebert
Address to the National Tuberculosis Association
May 31, 1965

Once upon a time at Philadelphia General Hospital, a frantic intern caring for a desperately ill patient submitted a request for consultation bearing the simple plea, "help!" A consultant responded to that request.

Treat your professional colleagues with respect; some day your patient's life (or possibly yours) may depend upon them. Your colleague's secretary may put you on hold, he may trump your diagnostic ace, your wives may compete socially, but when problems arise, your consultant will rise to the challenge.

In an emergency, your most valuable instrument is the telephone.

DOES YOUR PATIENT NEED A CONSULTANT?

Some cases require consultation—the diagnostic dilemma, the repeated therapeutic failure, or the restless patient who craves the reassurance of another opinion. When a builder remodels your home, he calls in consultants in plumbing, heating, and electrical repairs. No

179

builder or physician does all things well. Don't let false pride lead you into bungling cases beyond your training and experience.

The intelligent patient appreciates the value of specialist consultation. If another physician can provide superior care, you are morally obligated to suggest a referral. There are enough areas where your versatility outshines your consultant's erudition and plenty of waiting patients to keep you busy.

Consultation is a learning experience. Both the physician and his patient benefit from consultation, the patient gaining improved medical care and the referring physician garnering helpful hints to guide him when a similar problem is next encountered.

The specialist consultation should be arranged through your office. Liaison with consultants is the responsibility of the family physican, providing entry into our complex health-care system. If you scribble a few names on a prescription blank and leave the patient to battle an indifferent answering service or a protective secretary, your patient may soon feel he is trying to schedule an audience with the President himself, and the consultation you advised is short-circuited by faulty communication. Here's another way your aide can earn her salary: Explain the arrangements to be made, and allow her and the patient to use your private consultation room until a definite appointment has been scheduled.

REFERRAL ETIQUETTE

Live by the golden rule: Treat your consultant as you would have him treat you. Have respect for his busy schedule, requesting "emergency" consultation only in urgent cases, and allow consultations for chronic disorders to be arranged by appointment. You're sending the specialist your difficult cases; allow him time to figure them out.

The patient's history to date is of paramount importance in perplexing problems. Referring a patient "cold" forces the specialist to sort out information you may already have in your files. A preprinted form (Fig. 16–1) expedites referral and alerts the specialist to what you have done so far and what you have in mind. A complex case calls for a more extensive review of your records, supplemented by photocopies of pertinent laboratory data. In straightforward cases, such as a referral for tonsillectomy or hernia repair, I hand my patient the referral form, just as I would a prescription. In other instances, propriety dictates a sealed envelope, dispatched with the patient or mailed directly to the specialist.

ROBERT B. TAYLOR, M.D.
66 FOREST GLEN ROAD
NEW PALTZ, NEW YORK 12561

———

AREA CODE 914
TELEPHONE 255-5450

Date:_____

REQUEST FOR CONSULTATION

TO DOCTOR:_____

_____

_____

Telephone: _____

This will introduce my patient:

_____

Who is referred for:

_____

History to date:

_____

_____

_____

_____

_____

A report of your findings would be appreciated.

       Thank you.

             Robert B. Taylor, M.D.

Fig. 16–1. Form letter requesting consultation.

Referring unseen patients is rarely justified. Not all youngsters with head trauma require neurosurgical consultation, and most teenagers complaining of abdominal pain will survive without surgery. Before phoning your consultant, examine the patient yourself, using your own good judgment and experience to evaluate the necessity for referral. Hospitalizing all patients with chest pain and summoning a cardiologist would soon earn for you the rightful ire of your professional colleagues.

How to choose a consultant? "Mrs. Jones, Johnny has a hernia and should see a surgeon to have it repaired." I usually add the question, "Does your family have a favorite surgeon?" If they do, your problem is solved, but the usual reply is, "No, we don't doctor, I'll leave that up to you." Offer Mrs. Jones the names of two or more reliable surgical specialists in your area, but play fair with your consultants as well as with Mrs. Jones. When referring a nice easy hernia, don't forget the names of those loyal lads you call to cope with the 3 A.M. appendicitis attack. Send your paying patients to the same office you send your welfare clients.

Financial difficulties may mute the call for consultation. Don't let your patient's pleas of poverty influence your medical judgment. Your consultant, grateful for your more prosperous referrals, should happily accept your impecunious patients, usually allowing a lowered fee or none at all. But will he know the problem? Sure, you know that Mrs. Green exists on a minimal pension and have charged her reduced fees for years. But you also know she's too proud to tell the specialist, who lacks your long familiarity with your patient, about her financial woes. A telephone call can solve the problem: After Mrs. Green leaves your office, call the consultant (make this call yourself), alert him to Mrs. Green's marginal resources, and extend the hope that he will continue your policy of reduced fees.

Don't prejudice your consultant by labeling the patient "irritating", "crocky," or "malingering." Your patient is paying for an independent opinion, and even the purist specialist in his ivory tower may be influenced by implied or overt criticism by the family physician who, after all, knows the patient better than he. Remember, your judgments may be wrong. If you think Mrs. Jones dramatizes her complaints or Mr. Smith will make a startling recovery from his headaches as soon as litigation is terminated, keep these opinions to yourself. If they are valid, the specialist will confirm them without coaching.

Doctor Consultant, please talk to my patient. If you're on the receiving end of referrals, give my patient his money's worth. He's paying for an explanation of your findings and hopefully a plan of therapy. Don't short-change him with, "I'll discuss this with your family doctor, and he'll explain everything."

Report consultations in writing and do it promptly. Struggling in the boondocks, the family physician eagerly awaits the word from Mecca. A telephone call is expeditious, but all consultations should be reported in writing. A simple case? A tonsillectomy and adenoidectomy planned? Then complete your preprinted form and mail it out. A more involved case? Give the referring physician a full report. Not only will Mr. Patient contact his family physician within a few days to discuss the consultation, he will expect the family practitioner to have a full report when symptoms recur 6 months from now. Your telephone call may not be much help then.

DISTANT REFERRALS

"Doctor, I don't seem to be getting any better. Maybe I should go out to the Midwest Super-Clinic for a thorough examination." Unless you have a ready diagnosis and a foolproof plan of therapy, let him go. The aura of the big medical center, the ritual testing, and the penance of paying a whopping bill are all of therapeutic value.

The drama of the distant referral may hasten recovery as Mr. Patient finally becomes convinced that all possible avenues have been explored. How often I have seen patients return from a healing spa on the East Coast or the Midwest, clutching a voluminous tabulation of clinical data, a $2000 bill for services, and a prescription for the same Donnatal I advised 6 months before.

Regional medical center referrals are more to the point. They are usually arranged by a local consultant or yourself, and are necessitated by a complex medical problem beyond the scope of local facilities. Still, I undertake such a referral with some trepidation since it sets my patient adrift in a sea of white coats, searching for the beacon light of a little information. "Doctor, you sent my husband to the center at Gotham 3 weeks ago and nobody will tell me anything. Can you find out what's going on?" There he lies, a victim of team therapy, with medical care by committee. Where can the patient and his family get some straight answers? The solution lies with the original referring physician: Regional medical center referrals should be made by the local practitioner, speaking directly to one doctor at the center, transferring responsibility to his shoulders, with the implied obligation of keeping the patient, his family, and the local practitioner up to date. Someone must be captain of the ship, or no one will take responsibility for ordering a laxative. You, the referring physician, must choose the attendant physician and look to him for major decisions and reports.

WHEN PROFESSIONAL RELATIONS BREAK DOWN

Criticism of colleagues should be as rare as snowballs in the Sahara. Monday morning quarterbacks are always right. Symptoms change and physical findings develop as time passes. Of three consecutive physicians on a case, the last can usually make the diagnosis, blushingly outshining his predecessors. When tempted to be critical of a colleague (only in your thoughts, of course), ask yourself: "If I had handled the case *at that time*, might I not have come to the same conclusions and prescribed the identical therapy?"

The irate patient with fantasies of malpractice describes your colleague's callousness, ineptitude, and negligence. He's angry! He's sure he's been wronged and wants to act out his resentment. A wrong word, a pained facial expression, or an encouraging sigh can trigger litigation against a fellow physician. "I want to get that doctor. He shouldn't be allowed to practice medicine. He's going to pay for what he did." You try to reassure the irate patient that your colleague exercised his best professional judgment at the time. You might have handled the case the same way. But it doesn't work; he wants revenge. Give Mr. Irate Patient something to do: Instruct him to document his grievance in a letter to the Peer Review Committee of the County Medical Society, specifying times and places and quoting statements. Assure him that the Peer Review will study the case and reply to his complaint. Channel his anger in this direction and you've performed a valuable service for physicians and patients who, after all, inevitably foot the bill for professional liability insurance. The patient has vented his anger, the medical community has been alerted to a breakdown in professional relations, and Mr. Belli has been spared another courtroom drama.

References and Suggestions for Further Reading

1. Burdette J A: Can a GP make the grade on a big-name faculty? Med Economics 48:192–205, 1971

2. Cosby R S, Yett F A, Giddings J A, See J R, Mayo M: Physician-computer interaction as a clinical research technique. JAMA 218:1548–1551, 1971.

3. Fox R M: The Medical Report: Theory and Practice. Boston, Little, Brown, 1969.

4. Gaver J R: The Complete Directory of Medical and Health Services. New York, Universal, 1970.

5. Gloor R F: Family physician a partner in community medicine education. Am Fam Physician GP 3:165–168, 1971.

6. Hurst J W: The art and science of presenting a patient's problems. Arch Intern Med 128:463–465, 1971.

7. Jacobs A R: Emergency department utilization in an urban community: Implications for community ambulatory care. JAMA 216:307–312, 1971.

8. Menke W G: Professional values in medical practice. N Engl J Med 280:930–936, 1969.

9. Papper S: Attributes of a physician. Arch Intern Med 125:356–358, 1970.

10. Schwab J J, Brown J: Uses and abuses of psychiatric consultation. JAMA 205:65–68, 1968.

11. Toroey E F: Ethical Issues in Medicine. Boston, Little, Brown, 1968.

12. Tumulty P A: What is a clinician and what does he do? N Engl J Med 283:20–24, 1970.

17

So You Think
You Can Make a Living
as a Doctor

In the midst of your illness you will promise a goat, but when you have recovered, a chicken will seem sufficient.

African (Jukun) Proverb

The plumber charges $15 for a daytime house call; parts are extra. There are no disability forms for ailing fixtures, no discounts for indigent homeowners, and Washington has yet to dream up Plumbicare. No fancy office. No professional liability. Want your son to be a wealthy man? Forget medicine. Advise him to be a plumber.

THE INCOME-EXPENSES SEESAW

The doctor is a businessman; his success depends upon following sound principles of small business management. In a world full of 1.5 percent interest monthly charge accounts, fast-talking equipment salesmen, canny counselors, pitiful plaintiffs, "adjusted" Medicare payments, and patients who exhaust their monthly funds before paying the doctor's bill, treating scads of patients and charging fair fees just won't do. Month by month, the prudent physician must bolster his income and chip away at expenses, lest he spend his declining years carrying that little colored card from the Social Service Department.

Think I'm exaggerating? The HR10 (Keogh) Plan was enacted, not because of the federal government's solicitous concern for the welfare of physicians, not because of the entreaties of organized medicine, but because a nationwide survey revealed that a staggering percentage of sole proprietors spend their declining years on welfare. A sobering thought, Brother Sole Proprietor. And, Washington reasoned, welfare is expensive; let's let those poor devils provide for themselves.

Money comes and goes, you wave as it flies by. A whopping gross income looks impressive on paper, but it won't feed your family if it's exceeded by expenses. And however meager your net income, your federal silent partner is there to grab his share each April. To escape the indignity of poverty, the physician must employ business-like collection methods, cost accounting, income analysis, and every legal means to thwart the fiscal federal grab.

PROFESSIONAL OFFICE FEES

"Speck in cornea . . . 50 cents," accounting book entry, first fee as a practicing physician, quoted by Harvey Cushing in Life of Sir William Osler.

Here's where it all begins. John Patient visits you with a medical problem; his difficulty is resolved following an office call and a professional fee is due. What are the mechanics of this transaction?

The **charge slip** (Fig. 17–1) is your bill, prepared by the receptionist when John Patient enters the office. The charge slip accompanies Mr. Patient, acquiring notations by the physician, nurse, or technician along the way, until it is finally surrendered to the receptionist upon the patient's departure.

Your charge slips should be preprinted by a local stationer and should reflect the services available in your office. Annoying abbreviations should be avoided, and all information necessary to allow Medicare reimbursement should be included. The properly detailed charge slip is the patient's receipt, acceptable for income tax documentation. Duplicate forms with carbon or pressure-sensitive paper provide the patient with his receipt and your receptionist with a copy for posting. Here's a check list of items that should be included in your own charge slip:

1. Your name, address, and phone number
2. Date of the visit
3. Patient's name
4. Where to send the bill: patient, insurance company, or compensation carrier
5. Itemized charges, including laboratory, x-ray, therapy, injections, or other services commonly provided
6. Total charges
7. Amount paid: this is the receipt
8. When should the next appointment be scheduled?
9. A "reminder" line to alert your receptionist to address changes, new telephone numbers, the patient's desire for a flu shot reminder card next fall, or need for a gym excuse for Johnny's sprained ankle
10. Diagnosis: of vital importance to insurance clerks who will not reimburse Mr. Patient for his $8 office call before knowing whether he suffered a stroke or ingrown toenail
11. A notice that your charge slip is a valuable record, of potential interest to income tax investigators

Cultivate good charge-slip habits in your office. Every patient receives a charge slip even if he is known to have come for a "no charge" service, such as suture removal or cast check. All fees are entered on the charge slip when the procedure is performed: urine analysis, blood test, x-ray, electrocardiogram, office consultation. This rule includes every one at all times—nurse, technician, receptionist, and doctor. If John Patient visits briefly for blood tests in the morning and returns that afternoon for consultation and discussion of results, he gets two charge slips. If you wait to include the lab tests on his afternoon bill, they will probably be forgotten.

Number charge slips consecutively. Once upon a time, when I was young and naïve, I believed that charge-slip numbering was a waste of time and graphite. Then one week we compared charge-slip duplicates against the appointment book. Lo and behold, at least one charge slip daily was lost, strayed, or folded with the patient's prescriptions. However honest your patients, a pocketed charge slip means income down the drain. We now carefully number each slip, the first morning patient receiving No. 1. The final number of the day is a good measure of how hard you've worked, along with your sore back and aching feet.

Make your charge slip numbers inconspicuous. John Patient probably isn't interested in whether he's patient No. 2 or 35 that day, and your

Robert B. Taylor, M.D.
66 Forest Glen Road
New Paltz, N. Y. 12561

Office phone: 255-5450
Home phone for
   emergencies: 123-4567

Date: _____

Patient: _____

Bill to: _____

   Office visit _____ $_____

   Office surgery _____ _____

   Laboratory _____ _____

   X-ray _____ _____

   Electrocardiogram _____ _____

   Physiotherapy _____ _____

   Complete physical exam. _____ _____

   Injection _____ _____

   _____ _____

   _____ _____

                        TOTAL: $ _____

                AMOUNT PAID· $ _____

                     □ Dr.
Next appt.: □ Nurse _____

Reminder: _____

Diagnosis: _____

         Please keep this receipt for tax records

Fig. 17–1. Office charge slip.

daily patient volume need not become general conversation. Our numbers are penciled on the duplicate second sheet, unnoticed by all but the most inquisitive.

The diagnosis line can boomerang, particularly when your initial clinical impression is belied by subsequent events. Often it's best to keep the diagnosis general—abdominal pain, headache, infection. And, of course, you wouldn't inscribe "gonorrhea" for all the world to see. Older patients with chronic disease often have the same diagnosis each visit, copied from the face sheet (see Chapter 19).

Sometimes your aide forgets to add a polio vaccine or urine analysis charge. Catch the patient before he leaves the front desk, and the error is easily corrected. But once he's out the door, the bargain is sealed. The end-of-the-day realization that Mr. Patient wasn't charged for his penicillin injection should be forgotten in the interest of good doctor-patient relations. After all, it may cost you more than $2 worth of time to explain to Mr. Patient why you've added another charge to his bill. And you look pretty foolish.

The patient wants his money's worth. Make sure he knows he's getting it. Spend as much time as possible with the patient, often obtaining telephone consultations, dictating reports, and completing records while he is still in the room. Many hospital-based physicians sit in the patient's room to perform their time-consuming chart work.

"No charge" visits offset rampant rumors about money-hungry doctors. Mary Jones has a basal cell carcinoma of the face; little to do for her but arrange a visit to the plastic surgeon. Tommy Smith requires removal of the sutures the hospital put in last week, and Harry Brown needs a note certifying that his knee can withstand the rigors of high-school football practice. The little time and effort involved hardly justify a fee. I have at least one or two "no charge" office calls daily.

The patient's finances sometimes worry the doctor more than they should. Tempted to forego the throat culture or prescribe a less expensive antibiotic? Don't do it! If you ask your patient, he'd tell you, "Doctor, I just want to get well; a few extra dollars won't really make any difference." The most expensive medicine is the one that doesn't work. John Patient needs an electrocardiogram and *really* can't afford the additional fee? Then do it anyhow and forget the fee. In medicine, you won't be paid for everything you do.

Your fees are a fair measure of service to the patient. Don't be afraid to charge what you're worth. I still remember my first private practice patient, a youngster with an overwhelming aversion to higher learning who suffered disabling morning abdominal pains which disappeared dramatically as the school bus sped on without him. A counseling session and prescription for an antispasmodic solved the problem. But fresh from 3 years with the Public Health Service, I was quietly amazed that the mother considered my advice worth a $5 fee. But now I know about overhead and taxes; precious little of the $5 ever found its way into my bank account.

Discuss fees with your patients, particularly when undertaking prolonged or potentially expensive therapy. Mr. Patient may be reluctant to inquire but in the back of his mind a little voice is asking, "How much will all this cost?" Or there's the young couple who act embarrassed, "We'd like to bring our new baby to you if he's sick, Doctor, but get his check-ups and shots at the clinic." A few minutes of explanation, discussing the charges for well-baby care during the preschool period, will often gain the confidence of new parents and keep your young charge out of the clinic. What we don't need is more welfare patients.

Sky-high fees are self-defeating. Patients with modest financial resources can afford $5 to $10 office calls periodically; but if you assert your expertise with $50 consultation fees, colossal hospital bills, and relentless dunning, you may force your patient onto welfare. In the long run, modest charges to a private patient outweigh prestigious fees redpenciled by the County Social Service Department, and—most important—preserve your patient's dignity. Hippocrates said: "Sometimes give your services for nothing . . . and if there be an opportunity of serving one who is . . . in financial straits, give full assistance to all such. For where there is love of man, there is also love of the art."

ACCOUNTS RECEIVABLE

The family practitioner should **bill by family.** The name of each family member should be on the bill head, along with the address and phone number of the head of the household. Each charge is entered, including the date of the visit, the family member treated, the reason for the visit, and an itemization of specific charges. Payments are recorded as received, and a running total is kept. At billing time, the family ledger card (Fig. 17–2) is photocopied, then mailed with confidence and hope.

Sound too complicated? Think you'd rather bill each family member? I've seen it done, with statements rendered to 3-month-old Timmy Smith and the family with four children receiving six separate statements from one doctor. Uncle Sam loves the postage revenue, but the patient feels overwhelmed with the plethora of statements.

Separate certain account cards. Third parties confound the family billing scheme, necessitating separate accounts in the following cases:

1. Automobile accidents and other cases involving litigation require separate accounts. No matter how benign the injury appears, the first auto accident visit is posted on a separate account, filed under the "accident" heading. All professional fees relative to the injuries are recorded here, easily accessible when the plaintiff's lawyer informs you that the case is going to court tomorrow morning.

2. Workmen's Compensation fees are billed directly to the employer's insurance carrier and should never appear on your patient's family ledger card. Of course, you will adhere to the Workmen's Compensation Board fee schedule, and when Harvey Smith announces,

Robert B. Taylor, M.D.
66 Forest Glen Road
New Paltz, New York 12561
Telephone: 255-5450

Home Telephone:

123-4567

Mr. Thomas Smith
100 Main Street
Smalltown, Pennsylvania 00333

This statement includes:
1. Thomas
2. Mary
3. Thomas, Jr.
4. Anne
5.
6.
7.
8.
9.

ANY CHARGE OR PAYMENT AFTER THE LAST DATE WILL BE SHOWN ON NEXT MONTH'S STATEMENT.

DATE:	PROFESSIONAL SERVICES:	CHARGE:	PAYMENT:	BALANCE:
10 Mar.71	Office visit—Anne—tonsillitis——————— throat culture—————	8.00 3.00		11.00
Jun. 71	Office visit—Thomas, Jr.—sprained right ankle—————————— x-ray right ankle———————	8.00 15.00		34.00
10 Jun. 71	Office visit—Thomas, Jr.—recheck right ankle———————————	6.00		40.00
20 Jun. 71	Received on account———————————————		40.00	–0–
27 Sept.71	Office visit— Mrs. Smith—arthritis———————	8.00		8.00
22 Oct. 71	Received on account———————————————		8.00	–0–
3 Dec. 71	Office visit—Mr. Smith—viral flu—————————	8.00		8.00
31 Jan. 72	Office visit— Anne—2 year check up————————	8.00		16.00
4 Feb. 72	Received on account———————————————		16.00	–0–
10 Jun. 72	Office visit— Mr. Smith—hypertension————— urine analysis———————	8.00 2.00		10.00
12 July 72	Received on account———————————————		10.00	–0–

Please pay the last amount in this column: ➤➤➤➤

Fig. 17–2. Family ledger card.

"Doc. I've decided that this backache we've been treating for 3 weeks should be put over onto compensation," you grit your teeth and refigure the charges.

3. Your charges for hospital visits, although the patient's ultimate responsibility, are usually covered by at least one insurance company which requires an itemized statement uncluttered by other data. When your patient enters the hospital, begin a separate ledger card for him, headed "Hospital Care" and filed in a separate section of your Accounts Receivable. Upon the patient's discharge, the fees for hospital care are totaled, and the statement mailed promptly without waiting for your usual billing time.

4. Charges for nursing home care, almost always covered by Medicare, call for individual billing, even if more than one family member resides at the extended care facility. Medicare is geared to handle single-patient accounts, and combined family bills will be promptly rejected by a harried clerk happy to find an excuse to return Form SSA-1490 to "the supplier of services." Worse yet, she may "file" your statement, and you will receive a cordial form letter requesting another. Recent directives dictate that the reason for each nursing home visit be documented on the statement, and if you visit more often than monthly, be prepared to justify your visit in writing.

5. Insurance company statements are the fifth special category. Every day I answer several requests for information or perform an insurance medical examination, both fees payable by those giants of commerce and finance, the insurance companies. Of course, a bill is sent with the original report, but do you really know if all the bills are being paid? Maintain a separate ledger card for each of the insurance companies that refers patients and questionnaires to your office and record each transaction in the "charges" column. As payment is received, credit the account. When payments lag, mail a photocopy of your statement to the company. Keep these statements complete, including date, nature of service, patient, and the insurance company's case number.

Miscellaneous separate accounts are kept for camps, industries, and schools who pay for services. Since I live in a resort area, I care for several children's camps. I begin a new file each calendar year: Camp Monongahela: 1971, 1972, etc.; The Widget Company: 1971, 1972, etc.

Fee profiles color the billing picture. Bill Medicare the $7 you know they will pay (instead of your usual $10 fee), and before long your fee profile is fixed at $7 for that service. Then it's too late; pleas to Medicare to adjust your profile to realistic levels are answered by form-letter denials after a maddening 3-month wait. The solution? Bill your full fee to all third-party carriers (except perhaps the Workmen's Compensation Board), and let them make their "adjustments." Think your fee is justified, and the adjustment unfair? Then fight, with letters to your regional carrier and perhaps your Congressman. But be ready to document unusual services and extenuating circumstances.

Computer billing can update your collection system, with the speed of memory banks, the confusion of codes, and the snafus of mindless machines.

Proponents of computer billing cite the following advantages:

1. Accurate statements mailed monthly without delay
2. Precious office time is saved
3. Automatic aging of accounts, speeding payment
4. Comprehensive analysis of income to the practice

Opponents of computer billing, on the other hand, site the following shortcomings:

1. Duplication of services since your office aide posts receivables which are subsequently transferred by an operator to computer memory
2. Your records are out of the office, causing considerable confusion when old Mrs. Thompson calls to inquire about her bill.
3. The computer can't fill in forms correctly and produces jumbled data and inappropriate diagnoses
4. Income analysis is of little practical value to most small practices

Planning to give computer billing a whirl? Think carefully. Check the service's local references. The changeover period is expensive, frustrating, and time-consuming, justified only if the program eventually results in increased efficiency and reduced overhead. I studied the pros and cons of computer billing and finally decided to keep my records in my office, handy to the front desk when patients question charges. An efficient office accounting system, in my opinion, offsets the tenuous advantages of the computer and affords the priceless boons of a smiling face and cheerful voice.

Your **account cards** can spur collections daily, not only at billing time. Keep the account card file handy to the telephone, where your aide can cheerfully mention delinquent accounts when patients call. As Mrs. Jones checks out after her office visit, your aide can inquire, "I see you have not made a payment on your account recently. Wouldn't you like to pay something today?"

Billing day is harvest time. All accounts should be posted up to the minute. Want to avoid the first-of-the-month deluge, when your statement is buried in a stack of gas, electric, and telephone bills? Then make billing day the fifteenth of the month. During my first month in private practice, I ran out of money and sent out bills early. It worked so well that I still continue this practice, often receiving payment before Ma Bell's bill is even delivered.

COLLECTIONS

A physician who heals for nothing is worth nothing.

Baba Kamma
The Talmud

Payment while the patient is in the office means fewer statements to mail and fewer delinquent accounts. Methods vary from the doctor who charges no fixed fees, but allows patients to "pay what they think the services were worth" to the greedy gouger who demands cash payment in advance. Some offices have signs in the waiting room proclaiming the nebulous advantages to the patient of instant payment, with the veiled threat of fee increases if billing expenses increase overhead. Gimmicks and crass commercialism aside, the most reliable stimulus to prompt payment remains a cheerful aide who smiles and says expectantly, "That will be $10 today, please."

If you can't change a $20 bill, Mrs. Jones may charge her $10 fee, even though she planned to pay at the desk. As every small business has found, a supply of $1 and $5 bills is essential to conducting business. As much as $50 or $100 in small bills may be necessary in a big office, and the supply may need to be replenished every few days when accounts are deposited at the bank. Run short in between? Then keep a supply of 10 to 20 singles in your wallet for emergency use. Where to get the small bills? I quietly voice my displeasure with toll bridges and turnpike roads by presenting a large bill to the collector's outstretched palm. The change keeps my wallet well stocked with singles.

Transient patients depart and so does any chance of collecting your fee. Bend all efforts to collect charges while the patient is in the office, firmly hinting that out-of-town patients are expected to pay *now*. The patient has no money with him? Then offer your booklet of blank checks, purchased at a local office-supply store, handy for the transient patient to fill in the name and address of his bank, along with the amount of your fee.

Hippie patients bless you, but paying bills isn't their bag. Out goes your $8 statement, destined to carom from the post office "addressee unknown" or to disappear into the campfire of a local commune. Give it up, doctor; hippies don't pay bills—a philosophy consistent with instant gratification and disdain for responsibility. But sometimes, in a flush of gratitude, you may be rewarded with a few dollars while the hippie is still in the office.

Here's my hippie policy: "I know you're short on bread, but I can't afford to send you a small bill month after month. Pay me today what you can afford, and we'll call it even."

Reduced fee? Sure. Sometimes nothing at all. But in the long run, the pay-what-you-can philosophy has been financially successful and eliminates costly repeat billing of uncollectable accounts.

Slow payers need prodding. Every month a bill goes unpaid the likelihood of final satisfaction drops precipitously. The doctor's bill competes for attention with utility, department store, and servicemen's statements, most offering discounts for prompt payment and interest penalties for laggards. At present, medical ethics prohibit the doctor from using these two efficient collection devices, and your statement is often stuffed back in the unpaid-bill file once the checkbook runs dry.

Account aging describes the orderly succession of progressively more insistent collection notices accompanying monthly statements. On April 21, 1815, David Hosack wrote to one of his slow payers: "If the patient can abstain from unnatural indulgence he is readily cured by the means I have enumerated. A ten-dollar bill enclosed in your reply will be useful."

With the second unpaid statement, most offices begin to affix stickers, often color-coded. The first sticker respectfully calls the patient's attention to the statement, "which has apparently been overlooked." The next month's sticker may contain the word "delinquent" or "overdue." By the fourth month without payment, stronger measures are in order. Enclose a personal note (Fig. 17–3), alerting the patient that his bill has come to the attention of the bookkeeper, not merely a sticker-affixing machine. Enclose a color-coded reply envelope. No reply by month 5? Then a personal telephone call is in order, often best made in the evening by your part-time aide. Diplomacy is in order, and feedback from the patient can yield valuable information—an insurance mix-up, rank dissatisfaction, or even worse, overt anger with the threat of malpractice.

Fig. 17–3. Collection notice

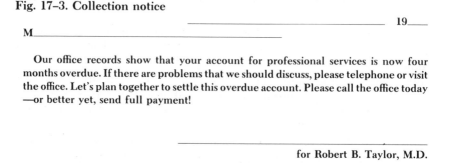

By the sixth month, when neither payment nor extenuating circumstances have been presented, the doctor must decide what to do about the account. Certainly, it would be a waste of time to simply mail further statements. You have three choices: Forget the bill and continue to treat the patient, turn the account over to a collection agency (who may not be as delicate as your aide has been), or dismiss the patient from your practice and write off the amount due. There's one final ploy: Send the patient a registered letter (Fig. 17–4) announcing that the account will be terminated either by referral for collection or retirement of the statement and that, in the future, you will treat the family on a "cash only" basis or not at all. Having to sign for a registered letter jolts the laggard, and the formality of notification often pries loose a few dollars.

Dunning is chastisement; make sure it's warranted. Each month, the doctor must review all statements receiving stickers, notes, telephone calls, and letters, wary that in a weak moment and unknown to his aide he may have made special arrangements with the patient. Thinking about referring an account for collection or dismissing a patient from your practice? Better review the clinical record carefully to make sure there is no medical basis for a claim of abandonment or retribution by litigation. Threaten your patient with legal action and he may respond in kind, given the opportunity.

Keep a written record of aged accounts, listing the month aging began, payments made, and written or verbal responses to notices. Your patient promised to pay $5 a week? Then write it down in the logbook. Some doctors record this promise on the ledger card so it faces the

Dear .... Date: ....

   Your family's account is now almost six months overdue. Perhaps there is some problem or question about the bill that we should discuss.

   In my office, my relationship with a family is terminated when a bill becomes six months overdue.

   Therefore, if this account is not settled within a month, I will, regretfully but permanently, withdraw my services as your family physician.

Robert B. Taylor, M.D.

Fig. 17–4. Final collection notice.

patient when his statement arrives each month. Once recorded, the patient's words can be read back to him in future conversations. "I don't remember any promise to pay by April." "Oh yes, sir, it's here in the book. You promised full payment."

Preprinted forms can speed payment when third parties are involved: The form should outline your office policy concerning auto accidents, school insurance, Medicare, and cases going to court (Fig. 17–5). The drudgery of preparing individual forms is avoided, and although the patient is referred to a single paragraph, he has before him an outline of your office's third-person policies. Many honest patients think an insurance premium negates their responsibility to the doctor. "Doctor, I sure hope you get *your* money from the insurance company." Answer? "We'll bill you and any insurance payment will be credited to your account. But in the end, my office will look to you for payment."

The term "collection rate" implies that the doctor doesn't always get paid. Realistic charges, prompt billing, efficient aging, and careful follow-up all help. Still, 2 to 5 percent of all fees remain uncollectable as thankless patients die, move away, or switch to a doctor with less efficient collection policies. Notwithstanding, your collection rate should be greater than 95 percent if the above tips are followed. A 100 percent collection rate shows you're pushing too hard, squeezing blood from stones, and probably swelling the welfare rolls. A collection rate of less than 90 percent is a symptom of illness in the practice, perhaps reflecting your guilt feelings, your aide's indolence, or an ignorance of how to make a living as a doctor.

No matter how devout his dedication, if the doctor's office doesn't show a profit, he won't be in the healing business long.

Robert B. Taylor, M.D.
66 Forest Glen Road
New Paltz, New York 12561

Telephone:
Office: 255-5450
Home (For Emergency Calls):
123-4567

DEAR PATIENT:

THE PARAGRAPH WHICH APPLIES TO YOUR SITUATION HAS BEEN CHECKED:

☐ MEDICARE (over 65) patients should save their office receipts. At the end of the year, if you have paid over $50 during the year, mail your receipts to Medicare to receive your refund. My office will be glad to help you fill in the form.

☐ SCHOOL INJURIES are covered by insurance which will reimburse you for part of your medical payments. When paying your bill, be sure to send along an insurance form.

☐ GROUP HEALTH INSURANCE (G.H.I.) will reimburse you for part of your medical payments. It is most convenient if you submit a signed form at the time of your office call.

☐ BLUE SHIELD pays the doctor all or part of his fee. The family is responsible for any difference between the bill and Blue Shield's payment.

☐ MEDIC-AID (welfare) is not accepted at this office. The family is responsible for all bills.

☐ AUTOMOBILE ACCIDENT AND LIABILITY CASES often take years to settle. Your medical bill should be paid monthly as treatment is rendered. Receipts will be provided as needed.

☐ REPORTS TO LAWYERS are prepared promptly, but only when the medical bill is paid up to date.

☐ MEDICAL REPORTS are not released from this office without the written authorization of the patient (or parent, if the patient is under age 21).

☐ PHOTOCOPIES of any existing record are made at no charge. However, for special reports, a charge for clerical services is added to your bill.

☐ INSURANCE FORMS are filled out only when the patient has completed his portion of the form. Please include any dates of disability or work missed. Forms are sent to the company unless you specify otherwise.

☐ FEES at this office are not determined by any outside agency. The family is responsible for any difference between my fees and payments by Medicare or an insurance company.

If you have any questions about billing or insurance problems, please call and we will try to work it out together.

Yours very truly,

Robert B. Taylor, M.D.

Fig. 17–5. Form outlining third-party policy.

WHERE DOES ALL THE MONEY GO?

Spending is the easy part: Write the checks and mail them out. But what is the stack of brightly colored checks buying?

The **overhead** in a general medical office should be 40 to 45 percent of the gross income. If it's more than that, you're paying nurses to knit, buying supplies you don't need, or practicing in a palace your income won't support. How about the doctor whose overhead is 30 percent? That's possible if he's a surgical specialist who makes his living in the hospital and maintains a small part-time office. But the family physician with a 30 percent overhead is probably skimping unnecessarily, giving injections himself, answering the office telephone, and laboring over insurance forms an aide could handle. Aides pay their way; so does the right equipment. Spend the money to update your practice, and watch your net income rise.

Salaries (including bonuses) should be 35 to 40 percent of your *overhead* costs—not of your gross income. Aides free the doctor to perform his specialized professional duties; they cope with phone calls, make appointments, render well-baby advice, administer therapy, give injections, and assume a vast array of responsibilities that ease the burden of office practice. My two registered nurses have their own schedule each day, including physical therapy, allergy shots, immunizations for foreign travel, blood tests, and dressing changes. They more than earn their salaries each week. Studies have shown that as the number of office aides increases, so does gross income.

Don't skimp on aides' salaries. Find out the hospital salary for nurses and match it. Your receptionist assumes duties far more taxing than a store clerk or telephone operator; pay her accordingly. Annual salary increments are in order, and your staff shouldn't have to ask for them. Their training is worth money to you—a discovery you'll make when Miss Efficiency leaves for a higher paying job in industry. Treasure your employees; reward them with respect, vacations, Christmas bonuses, and time off in emergencies. They'll repay you with loyalty, resourcefulness, and responsibility above and beyond the call of duty.

Your office: Should you rent or buy? Rent and the IRS forgives your monthly payments. Buy and you can deduct both the mortgage interest and annual depreciation. How about your area? Are professional offices available, handy to the hospital? Are rents reasonable? Is sufficient space available? How about parking and accessibility to public transportation?

When you plan your office, think big. Like aides, your office will more than pay its way. Think you need two examination rooms? Then plan three; you'll probably wish you had more. Storage space? There's never enough. Lavatories? One is mandatory, two better. The waiting room? Write down the number of people you will see each hour and multiply by 2. That's how many seats you will need, not counting the children's play area.

Plan to struggle along in your basement until you have enough money to buy or build? I wouldn't do it. Your local bank will be happy to lend you enough money to buy and equip your office. You're a first-rate credit risk. Use their money to build your dream office now. Don't wait until you are 50 years old and thinking about retirement.

Office supplies are the next biggest item in your professional budget. Your office supply salesman, calling weekly, earns a hefty commission on what he sells. But prices are often negotiable, and you only need to ask. Is there a discount for volume? Can I deduct 2 percent for payment by the tenth of the month? (Many major corporations live on that 2 percent.) Do you have a special this month—table paper, disposable syringes, examination capes?

Detail men representing major pharmaceutical corporations can often best the wholesaler's price by up to 25 percent. When they come around, stock up on orthopedic appliances and injectable steroids, saving precious overhead dollars.

Check your supply bill each month, including the item-by-item prices. Last month I was astonished to find I had been billed $20 for two Fleet enemas. A simple error: A clerk had read the item as two cartons and debited me accordingly. A careful check yielded a credit statement.

Office upkeep includes cleaning, lawn maintenance, plumbing, and electrical work. Are the servicemen your patients? Perhaps a "professional discount" can be arranged, reducing the monthly expenses for both.

Having trouble finding reliable maintenance personnel? Yes, cleaning women show up only half the time, and in my area at least, if you hire two servicemen, one will have a backache and the other will have to go home to get his tools. The solution? Deal with a professional service firm. Most localities have a professional office-cleaning service, professional maintenance services, and even an agency for part-time office help.

Cost accounting is familiar jargon to all businessmen. What does it mean? When you administer an injection of repository steroid and charge the patient $3, are you making a profit? Or, to put it another way, are you losing money? What does that bottle of steroid, that rib belt, that roll of plaster, or that urinary dip-stick cost you? There's only one way to tell: Examine your monthly statements carefully, mentally noting the item-by-item cost of supplies. What to charge? With inexpensive items, such as tetanus toxoid, DPT, vitamin B_{12}, and dressings, you are charging for service more than for the product. But with expensive items, the unit cost must be added to your service, and a good rule of thumb is to charge a *minimum* of twice your cost for expensive supplies. When you find a procedure or injection is unprofitable, it's time to raise the fee.

The "it's deductible" folly has been the ruin of many good men. The professional seminar in Outer Mongolia, the physical therapy machine with flashing lights that is used once monthly, and the gold-engraved patient-education booklet that nobody buys all cost money from the doctor's pocket, deductible or not. Resist the deductibility lures of insurance salesmen, once-a-year equipment venders, machine-addressed advertising folders, and 21-day South American "professional" cruises, and maybe you'll have a few dollars left at the end of the year.

The **cost of living** increases 6 percent annually, despite well-meaning attempts to freeze prices and wages. Wages, rent, supply costs, and maintenance charges all go up. Your fees must go up too. Each year, as you plan your aides' annual wage increases, dig out that written fee schedule you haven't glanced at in 12 months and refigure. Has the price of vaccines or dressings increased recently? Has your professional liability insurance gone up? If "yes" is the answer, then somehow, your fees must rise.

Many doctors leapfrog fees. First they charge extra for items that used to be "included"—throat culture, urine analysis, and pelvic examination. Once the higher total fee is fixed in the mind of the patient (and, more important, the doctor), the basic office fee is raised to cover the total, and the extras are again "included." The biggest stumbling block to sensible fee increases is the doctor's modest self-esteem coupled with his unfamiliarity with the actual cost of doing business.

Doctor, your patients are willing to pay to keep you in practice. Bill promptly, follow your accounts assiduously, and know your cost of doing business. Perhaps your income will match that of your plumber.

References and Suggestions for Further Reading

1. Cohen W J: The development and future of group practice prepayment plans. Public Health Rep 83:29–33, 1968.
2. Coulter D F, Llewellyn D J: The Practice of Family Medicine. Baltimore, Williams & Wilkins, 1971.

3. Darley W, Somers A R: Medicine, money, and manpower: The challenge to professional education. I. The affluent new health-care economy. N Engl J Med 276:-1234–1238, 1967.

4. Darley W, Somers A R: Medicine, money and manpower: The challenge to professional education. II. Opportunity for new excellence. N Engl J Med 276:1291–1296, 1967.

5. Ford A B: The Doctor's Perspective: Physicians View Their Patients and Practice. Cleveland, Western Reserve University Press, 1967.

6. Greco R, Pittenger R A: One Man's Practice: Effects of Developing Insight on Doctor-Patient Transactions. Philadelphia, Lippincott, 1966.

7. Hirsh B D: Business Management of a Medical Practice. St Louis, Mosby, 1964.

8. Millis J S: Is private practice dead? Calif Med 109:499–503, 1968.

9. Nourse A, Marks G: The Management of a Medical Practice. Philadelphia, Lippincott, 1966.

10. Roemer M I, DuBoid D M: Medical costs in relation to the organization of ambulatory care. N Engl J Med 280:988–993, 1969.

11. Rutstein D D: The Coming Revolution in Medicine. Cambridge, Mass, MIT Press, 1967.

12. Sheppard J D: The doctor's "business condition." Postgrad Med 47:202–207, 1970.

18

The Right Equipment Pays Its Way

The human body is the magazine of inventions, the patent office, where are the models from which every hint is taken. All the tools and engines on earth are only extensions of its limbs and senses.

Ralph Waldo Emerson
(1803–1882)

Once upon a time, the family doctor had an examination table in the parlor; he kept his records in his head, his accounts in his pocket, and his instruments in a little black bag. With the passing years, the doctor's "black bag" has ballooned to include the marvels of modern technology —x-ray, electrocardiograph, and photocopy machines—improving the physician's accuracy and productivity, but limiting his mobility. No longer can the physician, like his predecessor in days of yore, drive his buggy to the patient's home, set a fracture or repair a laceration, then collect his instruments and leave for home, dozing in the coachseat as the horse follows the familiar country road to the stable. Servants we are to electronic gadgetry, tolerated only because of the increased diagnostic accuracy and therapeutic effectiveness it allows.

YOUR MEDICAL OFFICE

The equipment and topography of your office should expedite the flow of patients and save you and your staff precious minutes and needless steps. Cramped quarters, obsolete equipment, and outdated methods lead to restless patients packed gluteus-to-gluteus in the waiting room.

The **waiting room** reflects the doctor's personality. Are you the modern type, who prefers imitation leather and chrome? Or perhaps you're traditional, offering a colonial decor. Whatever your decorating taste, the medical waiting room is no place for cast-off family-room furniture.

Furnish your waiting area with firm armchairs; overstuffed soft chairs entrap your elderly, obese, arthritic, or pregnant patients. Avoid love seats; rarely do two persons occupy that two-seater. Large sofas are colossal space-wasters; patients avoid sofa-sharing with strangers.

Provide enough seats. The average general office sees four to six patients each hour, and the waiting room should contain twice as many chairs as the anticipated hourly patient volume. A writing desk is helpful for patients with insurance forms to fill out. Miniature children's furniture keeps kiddies from competing with adults for seats, and during that once-a-week patient deluge, get out the extra folding chairs kept in the storage closet.

Music, supplied by an FM radio, prevents the ominous waiting room silence, lends a cheerful air, and most important, muffles the sound of your secretary's telephone conversation and your patient interview in the examination room.

The **examination room** is your workshop. The busy office will need three or perhaps four examination rooms—each completely stocked with diagnostic equipment and supplies. A wash-up sink is essential, and of course you'll have an examination table, writing desk, doctor's stool, and two chairs (for the patient and his omnipresent friend or mother). Tasteful framed prints relieve the clinical aura. Washable kitchen-type carpeting is aesthetically superior to tile, easier to clean, and more comforting to tired metatarsals.

Color-coded examination room doors help adults and children find their way around; resist numbering your examination room doors like doors in a bawdy house. "Mrs. Jones, after you've passed your urine specimen, go directly into the room with the green door." Here's a tip for the super-efficient office: Paint colored lines on the floor leading from the front desk to the color-coded examination room. "Johnny, you and your mother should follow the blue line to the room with the blue door."

The examination room desk reflects your practice methods. I like to sit while talking to my patients, and each examination room contains a 40-inch "salesman's" desk with a waterproof top and a file drawer for preprinted diets and forms. Most of my patients' visits begin and end in the examination room. If you consult in your consultation room and use the examination room only for the actual physical examination, a "stand-up" wall-hung writing desk may be in order. Whatever your desk choice, plan for rounded corners to prevent forehead lacerations in squirming infants. Arrange the furniture so the patient sits at your left, preferably with you between him and the door, allowing you a graceful exit when the interview is terminated.

The **treatment room** is the stage for your electronic wizardry. Here are found the x-ray machine (wall-mounted or portable), electrocardiograph, electrocautery apparatus, ultraviolet lamp, and other physical therapy equipment. Suture sets and plaster are kept here as well, to allow complete management of injuries without transporting the patient from examination room to x-ray room to treatment room. Necessarily oversized to house equipment, the treatment room should measure at least 12 by 16 feet.

The **laboratory** is really a catch-all room, housing the autoclave, incubator, refrigerator, and of course, the office laboratory equipment. Drug samples are usually stored here, preferably filed by usage in a 36- or 48-drawer file, appropriately labeled. Clean out your drug sample file every few months, discarding outdated medication and rarely used items.

If the lavatory and laboratory are adjacent, your local carpenter can construct a pass-through double door to spare your patient the embarrassment of wandering the hall clutching a bottle of warm urine and wondering who to give it to.

When designing your laboratory, remember that your nurses will be washing out surgical gloves, emesis basins, and urine specimen bottles; a drying rack over the sink keeps valuable counter space free of damp rubber gloves.

To store vaccines, throat culture plates, and medication samples that must be kept cold, you will need a larger refrigerator than you think. A tiny bar type won't do; 10 cubic feet of refrigerated storage space is minimum in a busy practice.

What else might your laboratory contain? A sink is necessary, preferably stainless steel. A chair can save your nurse's tired feet—there's probably nowhere else in the office for her to sit. Your double-locked narcotics cabinet is conveniently located here, although recent burglaries have proved the vulnerability of locks. Acting on the advice of my local supplier, I now keep only a few doses in the narcotics cabinet; the remainder are safely hidden in a less conspicuous place (still under lock and key). Finally, a corner of the laboratory, well away from chemicals, is the coffee spa, favored by the office staff and ubiquitous detail men alike.

Lavatories provide more than urine specimens. Hardly does Johnny enter the waiting room but he announces, "Mommy, I have to go potty." One lavatory is mandatory, but two are better; the second prevents mishaps due to occupied facilities and saves precious minutes when a urine specimen is needed on a busy day. At least one lavatory should be handy to the waiting room, so the patient with a distended bladder need not wander through your treatment area, looking for the comfort station. Paper towels prevent cross infection, but may find their way into your plumbing unless a large waste basket is available in the lavatory. Many physicians stack disposable plastic urine specimen bottles on the toilet lid, rather than handing them to the patient upon dispatching him for a specimen.

Hallways are often space-wasters and cause bottlenecks if narrow or ill-lit. Put your hallway space to use: A wide (8-foot) hallway can contain scales for adults, a weighing station for infants, storage cabinets, and a nurse's station for administration of injections. If your laboratory is cramped, place your refrigerator in the hallway. Here's where you store your wheelchair, essential if you treat acutely ill or injured patients (and don't we all?). Since it's probably your only unobstructed 20-foot area, the hallway should contain your visual acuity chart. Spotlight illumination of the Snellen chart is necessary, and because hallways usually lack windows, extra lighting is needed here.

The **business office** is never big enough. Plan sufficient space to house the files of at least 5000 patients (see Chapter 19), the necessary office equipment, ledger cards, and the multitude of odds and ends needed to run a busy office. Plan an extra work area for part-time help during busy periods; your nurse can sit here when she writes immunization reminders. Store typing supplies handy to the front desk, so your aide doesn't leave her post each time she needs an envelope. As your practice grows, so will your storage needs; plan enough room.

Sitting at her desk, your aide's view commands the waiting room. Areas hidden from her view mean overlooked patients, sitting quietly, wondering why their names aren't called. As each patient enters the office, the aide acknowledges his arrival and hands the record to the nurse. Within arm's reach your aide should have telephone, appointment reminder file, and account cards. This arrangement requires considerable counter space; an excellent solution is a U-shaped front desk.

The **consultation room** is the doctor's private retreat, handy to the back door and the business office. Here is his medical library, personal correspondence, and private telephone line for emergencies. Distraught relatives, prospective employees, and visitors are interviewed here. On busy days, the consultation room serves as an isolation area. Memos for the doctor's attention are left on his desk and dispatched as time allows. When your rooms are jammed with elderly matrons tugging on their corsets, hold your end-of-the-visit discussions here, freeing an examination room for a waiting patient.

How much space is required? For the busy family practice, 1500 square feet is about right, allowing ample room size and enough space for smooth traffic flow. The 1000-square-foot office may creditably serve the specialist seeing 6 or 8 patients in an afternoon, but a busy GP, caring for 30 to 50 people daily, needs room. The floor plan shown in Figure 18-1 was developed following months of study and reams of trial-and-error drawings, and finally built in 1968. The floor plan has the following advantages:

1. A large waiting area visible from the front desk
2. A sound buffer (the cellar stairway) between the waiting room and nearby examination room
3. Two identical examination rooms with wall-hung sinks
4. A wide hallway used as a work area
5. A large treatment room, allowing concentration of equipment in one area
6. Two lavatories, one handy to the waiting room
7. A laboratory with plenty of counter space and a pass-through door to an adjacent lavatory
8. A side door entry for emergency patients and unobtrusive exit of the physician
9. A large business area, overlooking the waiting room, with ample wall space for chart filing
10. A direct line of vision from the front desk to the laboratory and doctor's consultation room
11. An outdoor sheltered area where patients can await the doctor's arrival

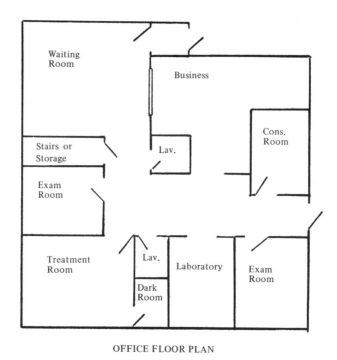

OFFICE FLOOR PLAN

Fig. 18–1. Floor plan for a 1500-square-foot office.

12. Examination room doors hung to hide the gowned patient on the
examining table

DIAGNOSTIC EQUIPMENT

The **electrocardiograph,** indispensable in the diagnosis of arrhythmias
and myocardial infarction, belongs in every family physician's office.
With training, your office nurse can record the tracing within a few
minutes. Read the EKG yourself. Feel a little shaky about your readings? Then brush up by reviewing standard texts or taking a correspondence course, such as "Difficult Electrocardiographic Diagnosis," given
by the Department of Post-Graduate Medical Education, University of
Kansas Medical Center, Kansas City, Kansas, 66103 (approved for 15
postgraduate hours by the American Academy of Family Physicians). A
local cardiologist will be happy to review your most puzzling tracings.

Crossed leads can cause apparent abnormalities. Instruct your aide to check lead I with each tracing. The P wave and QRS complex in lead I should be upright; if they are inverted, suspect incorrect electrode placement.

Paper is cheap. Instruct your nurse to record at least five complexes with each lead, perhaps including a long lead II in a patient with an arrhythmia.

Trouble shooting a malfunctioning electrocardiograph can cause gray hair, especially on busy days. Before summoning a serviceman, check the following: Is the wall outlet connection firm? (If the plug is two-pronged, withdraw the plug and reinsert it.) Is the service wire connected firmly to the set? Are the leads attached properly? Has a fuse blown? Did the last user insert the paper properly? Is the stylus heat too high? Have you tripped a circuit breaker on the outlet?

None of these? Then better call for help.

The office **x-ray** is indispensable to the busy family physician, especially if his office is located more than a few minutes from the hospital. The office x-ray unit costs about $4000 to $5000 and should pay for itself within a year. A portable x-ray unit works well, but a wall-mounted unit, allows more uniform technique and less radiation scatter. If the x-ray machine is installed in a multipurpose treatment room, the doctor may decide, as I did, to substitute for the Bucky table an ordinary wooden treatment table which is also useful for casting and repairing lacerations. Those few cases requiring Bucky plates can be accommodated with a grid-front cassette.

The darkroom can double as a projection booth, saving valuable floor space. Using leaded glass, which transmits light but not x-rays, your carpenter can construct a double window that allows the passage of sound but blocks x-rays (Fig. 18-2). The light-tight door of the projection window can be closed when film developing is in progress.

X-ray film is available in various sizes, but for the general office, only 14- by 17-inch and 10- by 12-inch plates are necessary. Lead blockers can be used to reduce exposure size when necessary.

Lead lining is important, and trust your county health office to check your installation. The x-ray room must be lead-lined on all walls where the danger of x-ray exposure threatens persons in nearby rooms. Unless there is a building within 50 feet, exterior walls need not be leaded. Ceilings and floors must be lead-lined only if the floor below or above is occupied. Interior walls, including doorways, should be lined to a height of 7 feet with lead foil at least 1/32 inch thick. Overlapping lead linings are installed in the door casing. Since the leaded door may weigh more than 100 lb, multiple heavy-duty hinges will be needed.

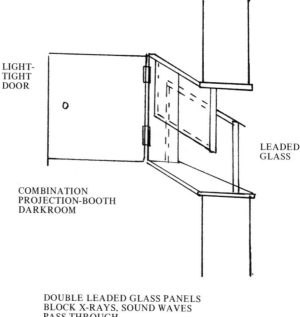

LIGHT-
TIGHT
DOOR

LEADED
GLASS

COMBINATION
PROJECTION-BOOTH
DARKROOM

DOUBLE LEADED GLASS PANELS
BLOCK X-RAYS. SOUND WAVES
PASS THROUGH

DARKROOM–PROJECTION BOOTH WINDOW

Fig. 18–2. Window for combination projection booth and darkroom. Double leaded-glass panels block x-rays but allow sound waves to pass through.

The electrician should install a red warning light over the door outside the x-ray room to alert the staff that the unit is in use.

The collimator limits unnecessary radiation to the patient and allows accurate centering of x-rays. In youngsters, supplement the collimator with a lead apron.

When you perform chest x-rays on modest matrons, a short gown covers the chest and an examination sheet around the waist held in place with a Kelly clamp preserves dignity.

Read your own x-rays. With prompt developing, the wet print is available within 10 minutes after exposure. Be sure to review the film a second time once drying is complete. Send difficult-to-interpret films to the hospital radiologist for consultation and a written report.

PHYSICAL THERAPY EQUIPMENT

Some young doctors scoff at physical therapy. "Witchcraft," they call it; but with the passing years, most physicians learn the value of judicious physical therapy.

Whirlpool, like most other physical therapy modalities, delivers heat. The motion of water provides gentle massage, enhancing the therapeutic value of heat. Useful in treating athletic injuries, whirlpool treatments speed recovery and emphasize to the young athlete that he is not yet well enough to risk his limb for the glory of his local secondary school.

Hot packs, claim the purists, are the best method of applying heat, the moisture enhancing penetration. Inexpensive and adaptable to difficult areas inaccessible to diathermy and ultrasound, hot packs are often applied using Hydrocollator pads. A thin coating of mineral oil or Dermassage protects the skin. Avoid excessive wetness, which may result in painful burning, the most common complication of this mode of therapy.

Ultrasound generates high-frequency (700,000 to 1,100,000 cps) sound waves, inaudible, but capable of penetrating tissue. The indications for ultrasound include arthritis, bursitis, radiculitis, painful injuries, fibrositis, and neuroma. Caution your nurse not to use ultrasound near the heart, eyes, or reproductive organs and not to use it on pregnant women or patients with cancer. Capable of interfering with bone growth in children, the use of ultrasound is probably best restricted to adults. Ultrasound is usually prescribed as 5-minute treatments at an intensity of 0.5 to 2.0 watts per square centimeter, repeated daily or several times weekly.

Here's a tip you should learn from a book rather than by experience: Ultrasound treatment over the carotid sinus can lead to syncope.

Diathermy is another method of delivering heat to deep tissues, increasing circulation and relieving pain. In my practice, diathermy is rarely a first-choice treatment method. I find hot packs and ultrasound more effective. A diathermy treatment ties up an examination room for 20 minutes and lacks the comforting human hand on the ultrasound applicator.

The indications for diathermy are the same as those for ultrasound—conditions calling for heat. The diathermy head is positioned with a spacing bar, usually 3 to 5 inches from the affected area. The physician should prescribe the spacing distance, percent of power, and treatment duration for each case; a common prescription is a 20-minute treatment at 80 percent of power with a spacing distance of 4 inches.

Diathermy should not be used in malignancy, infection, over ischemic areas, over edematous tissue, and over growing bone. Metallic implants or adhesive tape on the skin may absorb heat and cause painful burns.

Diathermy has two major advantages. Patients with cervical sprain, in whom ultrasound therapy may produce syncope, have not experienced adverse reactions to diathermy treatments in my office. Although diathermy requires 20 minutes for administration, its use frees the nurse to perform other duties; the patient is left with a bell to ring and is instructed to summon the nurse if the treatment area becomes hot.

Ultraviolet phototherapy should be used more often; most doctors are ignorant of its advantages. Beguiled by antibiotics, we have allowed the bactericidal and fungicidal benefits of ultraviolet light to fall into disuse. Ultraviolet therapy is useful in dermatophytosis, impetigo, infected ulcers, psoriasis, and infected diaper dermatitis. "Incurable" tinea pedis has been eradicated following ultraviolet phototherapy.

The eyes of patient and operator must be shielded (Fig. 18-3). Whether you use the higher wattage cold quartz or the lower wattage filament-activated mercury vapor lamp, your unit should be calibrated on normal skin before it is used on a patient. Treatment duration varies from a few seconds to 5 minutes, depending upon the manufacturer, and treatment is usually repeated every day or two until the lesion clears. The course of therapy should rarely exceed 3 weeks. Although supplementary topical medication may be used, it should be removed prior to phototherapy, because ultraviolet light penetrates foreign matter and tissue poorly. In most cases, a mild erythema will be noted, enhancing the skin's antibacterial and antifungal activity.

Ultraviolet therapy is contraindicated in pellagra, xeroderma pigmentosum, systemic lupus erythematosus, porphyria cutanea tarda, erythropoietic protoporphyria, and photodermatitis.

Help your aides by typing full instructions for the use of each therapeutic device on a 3- by 5-inch card and taping the card to the machine. Include danger signals and contraindications.

BUSINESS OFFICE EQUIPMENT

Doctor, you wouldn't consider riding to your patient's bedside in a horse-drawn buggy, examining his chest with a monaural stethoscope,

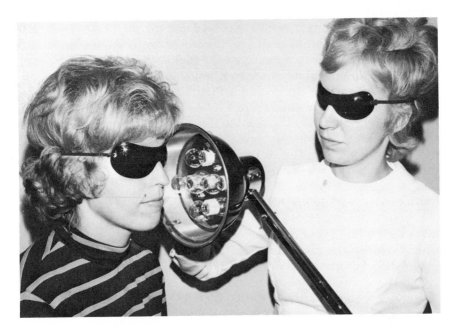

Fig. 18–3. Ultraviolet phototherapy.

and treating him by cupping. Archaic? Right! Then you certainly shouldn't ask your aide to struggle with an outmoded manual typewriter, carbon paper, and a dime-store pencil sharpener. If your daily income doesn't require the services of an adding machine, your practice needs help. Along with up-to-date diagnostic equipment, the modern medical office needs the machines of modern business.

The **electric typewriter** is the backbone of your business office. The days of handwritten professional communications are gone, along with the art of penmanship. Except for prescriptions, correspondence leaving your office should be typed. That includes referral slips, gym excuses, insurance forms, and medical reports. Saddle your secretary with the old portable you used in medical school, and it's a toss-up whether she'll develop arthritis of the fingers or quit first.

Respect your aide's professional ability and provide her with the proper tools. Office-quality electric typewriters cost $300 to $500 and are worth every penny. Perhaps your aide has previous experience or a strong preference. Let her help you choose, and be careful to deal with a supplier who will provide service after the sale is made.

A **photocopier** is as indispensable as the electric typewriter. Used almost hourly in a busy office, the photocopy machine takes center stage at billing time, as ledger cards are copied and the duplicate enveloped and mailed. Duplicate reports and insurance forms are a snap.

I began practice with an inexpensive photocopy unit, buying paper at 5 cents a sheet, adding solutions like a mad chemist, and eventually being rewarded with damp copies that faded when exposed to light. Over the years, I've worked up to Xerox—the Cadillac of the industry. I've tried other machines, including the one at the hospital, and none are in the same league. My present model costs $600 annually, but repairs are included. The Xerox photocopier can use any 20-weight paper, considerably less expensive than chemically treated sheets or rolls of paper.

An **electric adding machine** costs about $100, and if you can't afford this, you're in trouble. Built to last for years, the adding machine has many uses: adding your daily deposit, balancing your checkbook (here's where you use the minus key), and helping junior with his math.

Dictating equipment is optional. If you write few letters, and your secretary can read her shorthand once it gets cold, you may not need it. Some secretaries actively dislike dictating equipment, while other happily plug in the earphones and tune out the world.

I couldn't get along without it. I use a portable Norelco dictation set, and my secretary has a matching office model. Reports that would take hours to inscribe by hand roll trippingly off my tongue. I drive my car or sit at home dictating ideas or instructions as they come to mind—patients seen, memos, chores to do, servicemen to call, and reports to complete. I enter the office in the morning, hand my secretary the tape, and the finished work is on my desk by the day's end.

The **electric pencil sharpener** is a pleasant, inexpensive luxury. Show your secretary you care. Get her one for Christmas.

An **office intercom system** eliminates shouting down the hall. A commercial intercom system can also pipe canned music into your examination room, but some patients express suspicion that conversations may be overheard. More practical is the telephone intercom line, using your examination room phone extension. Here's where you can save some money. A station-to-station intercom set-up costs about $2 *per station* monthly. On the other hand, a single open intercom line to all stations costs only $2. If you have six telephone outlets, as I do, you can save $10 monthly by installing your own buzzer system. Your electrician can install a room-to-room buzzer arrangement, or better yet, a single buzzer audible throughout the office can alert the staff to pick up the intercom: A single buzz calls the receptionist, two the nurse, and three the doctor. A short buzz followed by a long can signal the nurse to enter the doctor's examination room, breaking up a long-winded monologue.

References and Suggestions for Further Reading

1. Fields W S, Spencer W A: Stroke Rehabilitation: Basic Concepts and Research Trends. St Louis, Green, 1967.
2. Friedman H H: Outline of Electrocardiography. New York, McGraw-Hill, 1963.
3. Jackson W: Dose assessment in diagnostic radiology. Br J Radiol 40:301–308, 1968.
4. Levine S N: Advances in Biomedical Engineering and Medical Physics, vols I, II. New York, Wiley, 1968.
5. Meschan I: Roentgen Signs in Clinical Practice. Philadelphia, Saunders, 1966.
6. Saenger E L: Radiologists, medical radiation and the public health. Radiology 92:-685–699, 1969.
7. Schreiber M H: Indications and Alternatives in X-Ray Diagnosis. Springfield, Ill, Thomas, 1970.
8. Williamson P: Office Procedures. Philadelphia, Saunders, 1960.

19

It's Right Here in the Record

Good God! This is a dreadful record. You can't tell anything about the patient. You can't tell whether he's married, single, or Australian!

> Sir F.M.R. Walshe
> *Comment on a case record written by an Australian*
> *clinical clerk, National Hospital, London, 1930*

Within 30 seconds, you should be able to locate any fact in any record of any patient in your practice. Needless minutes spent rummaging through ill-filed reports and deciphering cryptic notes represent unproductive office time. Quickly accessible, easy-to-read medical records can increase practice productivity, and the doctor can spend those otherwise wasted minutes treating patients.

Your medical records are the diary of your practice—the hour-by-hour, day-by-day story of your professional life. Moreover, each folder tells the story of one patient's injuries and illnesses, perhaps beginning with his neonatal visit and continuing through tonsillitis, appendicitis, school physical examinations, football injuries, college physical examination, premarital examination, hernia repair, cholecystectomy, hypertension, angina, and heart attack.

Until our generation, the physician's medical records were inviolable. Soon, the incursion of government into the practice of medicine will send inspectors into your office. Groping for yardsticks to measure the "quality" of medical care, auditors seize upon the medical record as indicative of the physician's professional competence. Compile your records carefully. Big Brother is watching.

THE ORGANIZATION OF GOOD MEDICAL RECORDS

Do you know who your patients are? The doctor with a good tight practice does. As each family enters the practice, a roster card (Fig. 19-1) is completed, listing names and birth dates of all family members and the family's address and telephone number.

Head of Household ..... Thomas Albert Smith (Sr.) .....

Address ..... 100 Main Street .....

..... Smalltown, Pa. .....

Telephone: ..... 123-4567 ..... Date of birth: ..... 8/4/32 .....

All other family members on this account:

	NAME:		DATE OF BIRTH:
1.	Mary Louise Smith	—	2/3/33
2.	Thomas Albert Smith Jr.	—	9/12/58
3.	Anne Marie Smith	—	1/31/70
4.		—	
5.		—	
6.		—	
7.		—	

Fig. 19–1. Patient roster card.

Keep this card file near the telephone and account posting tray to facilitate identification. Is Johnny Jones the son of Harry Jones or of Frank Jones? Memory may fail you but your patient roster won't. "Check" the patient's name once a file folder is completed, saving needless steps to determine whether Johnny already has a folder.

Each patient must have his own folder. In the days before dial telephones and television, a family's records were kept in a single folder; in-laws, cousins, and children were added as they appeared on the scene. In those days retrieval was simple; the doctor kept most records in his head. With the emergence of interested third parties—insurance companies, government agencies, and compensation carriers—demands for detailed information convinced most physicians of the caprice of memory. Now, the family folder is an anachronism, important only to medical historians.

Middle names become important as your practice grows. In my small town three of us share the same first and last name. Jones, Smith, and

Brown are notoriously common, but less common surnames abound in various regions of the country. The habitual inclusion of the patient's first, middle, and last names can prevent record mix-ups.

Birth dates identify patients like fingerprints: Insurance companies always identify the patient by name and birthday. Include these dates on your patient roster card and clinical record. A quick check discloses that little Timmy Brown wasn't born in 1899. Individual file folders are unnecessary for summer campers, vacationing tourists, itinerent workers, and industrial employees, unlikely to return for repeat visits. Each transient visit should be recorded on an individual progress sheet, filed by category, with new folders added annually: Widget Company employees, 1972; Overlook Hotel guests, 1972; Camp Monongahela, 1972; Migrant farm workers, 1972.

The **face sheet**, a concept borrowed from hospital records, contains pertinent information about the patient, including name, date of birth, address, head of the household, telephone number, sex, race, and marital status (Fig. 19-2). A list of the patient's allergies appears here, as does a summary of chronic illness, past medical history, and family history. The handy immunization record helps you keep your patient's shots up to date.

Progress notes are recorded on firm lined paper. Light cardboard prevents dogeared pages and permits both sides of the page to be used. My progress notes contain the doctor's name and address, front and back, to identify the source of records when they are photocopied. Transient records are recorded on progress sheets, filed by hotel, camp, and so forth.

The **laboratory sheet** is a page of light cardboard on which are taped those small lab slips that would otherwise clutter your files.

Letter-sized electrocardiograph, x-ray, and consultants' reports are filed behind the lab sheet, arranged in chronologic order.

Color-code your sheets for easy retrieval: The face sheet can be buff-colored, the progress notes white, and the lab sheet green or blue.

What **type of folders** should you use? Clip-in folders hold reports in an orderly sequence and are particularly useful in clinics where handling by multiple aides may result in shuffled pages. But clip-in folders require removal of all sheets to extract a single report—a disadvantage when one sheet is to be photocopied. Flat folders without clips save filing space and facilitate rapid removal of single items.

Medical record entries should support your clinical diagnosis and justify the treatment prescribed (Fig. 19-3). While dressing changes and routine immunizations necessitate only short entries, more difficult problems require elaboration. Pay particular attention to automobile accidents, Workmen's Compensation cases, and complicated clinical problems.

Robert B. Taylor, M.D.
66 Forest Glen Road
New Paltz, N.Y. 12561

NAME:_____Thomas Albert Smith, Jr._____

DATE OF BIRTH:__9/12/58_____   TELEPHONE:__123-4567_____

ADDRESS:____100 Main Street_____

____Smalltown, Pa._____

BILL TO:____Thomas A. Smith, Sr._____

ADDRESS:__Same_____

OCCUPATION:____Student_____

INSURANCE:__Blue Shield and Blue Cross_____

Ⓦ N O   M Ⓢ W D   Ⓜ F

Drug Allergies: IMMUNIZATIONS:

1.   Penicillin   DPT:_11/3/58_ DT:_7/10/68_ FLU:_____
                                      12/3/58
2.   1/4/59
                                      11/6/60
3.   8/10/63

Chronic Illness:

1. Rheumatic heart disease   TET. TOX.:   MEASLES:
                              (injury)2/1/70   12/4/69
2.

3.   MUMPS:
                                                 1/3/70

Past Illness and Surgery:

1.1960-Right inguinal hernia   VAC.:_11/4/69_ SALK:_____ SABIN:_11/3/58_
        repair   1/4/59
2.1968-Acute rheumatic fever   3/6/59
                                                                   11/6/60
3.   8/10/63
                              OTHER: 7/10/68
4.   8/3/69 Tine TB Test-Negative
                                                               RUBELLA:
5.   2/4/71

6.

Family Illness:

1. Father- Hypertension

2. Mother- Rheumatoid arthritis

3. Sister- Congenital heart murmur

4.

Fig. 19–2. Office record face sheet.

bert B. Taylor, M.D.
Forest Glen Road
ew Paltz, N. Y. 12561

Name ..Thomas Albert Smith, Jr.............................

Address ....100 Main St.   Smalltown, Pa..................

3 June 71 Fell in gym at Smalltown Central School at 1:30 PM today.
            Complains of pain in right ankle.

            No history of previous right ankle injury.

            Physical examination: cannot bear weight on right ankle.

            Ligaments appear intact. Strong right dorsalis pedis pulse.

            Right ankle x-ray: AP, lateral, and stress view with left

            ankle for comparison: No evidence of fracture or dislocation.

            Ankle mortise intact

            Diagnosis: sprain right ankle

            Treatment: 3 inch Ace bandage.

                    Crutches with no weight bearing
                    Aspirin 10 grams every 6 hours for pain

                    Elevation

                    Ice packs 1 hour 4 times daily for 3 days

                    No physical education in school for 6 weeks

            Return in 1 week

                              R. Taylor MD

10 June 71 Recheck right ankle:

            Complains of little pain.

            Physical examination of right ankle: Minimal swelling,

            tenderness, and ecchymosis. Good stability of joint.

            Diagnosis: sprain right ankle, responding well.

            Treatment: Continue 3 inch Ace bandage during daytime
                    hours for 10 days.

                    Warm saline soaks 1 hour twice daily for 5 days.

                    Limited weight bearing for 1 week,

                    then full weight bearing.

            Return if worse or if not well in 2 weeks.

                                R. Taylor MD.

Fig. 19–3. Medical record entries on progress sheet.

Although not necessary at each follow-up visit, a complete record entry should follow the clinical evaluation of any new disorder. A good record entry includes:

1. Date of the visit, including time of day
2. Why and how the patient came to you (visiting from out-of-town? brought by ambulance? covering for another doctor?)
3. Chief complaint and duration of symptoms (in accident cases, record exact time, place, and nature of injury)
4. History of the present illness, including all described symptoms and negative responses to questions
5. Pertinent past medical history, family history, and social history
6. Physical examination, with details of significant positive and negative findings
7. Laboratory tests (include results of x-ray, electrocardiography, urine analysis, and blood tests)
8. Diagnosis (try to be consistent here; changing your diagnosis from visit to visit confuses aides and insurance adjusters)
9. Plan of management (include medication, physical therapy, and work restrictions)
10. Prognosis (state your best estimate of partial and total disability)
11. Plan of follow-up (will the patient return in 2 days or 2 weeks?) Minimum advice should include the admonition to return if worse or within a specified time if not recovered.

Here's a clever filing tip: Each of us has a few patients with unusual conditions (rheumatoid pleuritis or subclavian steal syndrome). When you find a useful article concerning the illness, tear it out and file the original article in your patient's chart.

Your patient's clinical record must not become cluttered with non-medical trivia. Keep your records to the point by eliminating outdated account cards, old check stubs from insurance companies, and personal correspondence.

Entries in your clinical records must reflect your professional demeanor. Witty quips and personal invective have no place here. Phrases like "acute exacerbation of chronic crockism" could cost your professional liability insurance carrier thousands of dollars should your clever comment prove inaccurate. Include nothing in your records that would cause embarrassment if read back to you in court.

RECORD STORAGE

File your clinical records carefully. You may want to find one some day. That 30-second retrieval time I mentioned includes locating the patient's folder, ideally without opening a single drawer.

Open-stack filing is the modern way. The old pull-out medical file wastes space and motion. Think about it. The actual space occupied by a pullout file is the number of square feet covered when a drawer is *opened*, twice the area needed to store the same number of charts in open stacks. With open-shelf filing, a short aide can locate charts at eye level or above; try that with pullout files. Hardboard dividers separate sections of the alphabet. Use one divider for every 25 to 50 folders.

Color-coded folders speed refiling and prevent lost charts. Misfile a record? With color-coding you need search only three letters of the alphabet. Color-coded folders are available (but often on special order) at your local stationery store or can be mail-ordered from the Colwell Company, 201 Kenyon Road, Champaign, Illinois, 61820. The following is a workable color-designation scheme that I have used in my practice, coming out a little light on black folders (black is a depressing color anyhow) and slightly heavy on light green (a nice soothing hue):

Brown	A K U
Orange	B L V
Light Green	C M W
Yellow	D N X
Red	E O Y
Dark Blue	F P Z
Black	G Q
Pink	H R
Dark Green	I S
Gray	J T

Insist that your secretary block print the patient's name; last name first, then first name, and middle name or initial. Typed labels affixed to the folders are better. Handwritten names can result in misfiling.

Tag the site of a removed folder. Tracer cards are used in large institutions to identify the present location of the record and mark the spot for refiling. My small office, where records never leave the building, uses the simple expedient of pulling the adjacent record out about 1 inch to mark the locus for speedy replacement. My secretary dreamed up this filing tip, and I spent 2 weeks pushing folders back where they belonged, before she told me what she was doing. It saves minutes. Try it.

Where to file the unfilable? The "odd file" contains 26 alphabetical folders for orphan reports. Here rest data concerning patients who don't yet have file folders and medical reports concerning patients transferring to my practice from another area. Review the odd file monthly and find homes for the orphans.

How about numbered charts? I tried it once. Those charts were all business, easily assimilated by data processing and easy to refile, but in time the disadvantages outweighed the good points, and I abandoned numbered charts. Try as he might, the patient could never remember his number. So two motions were needed to find the folder: first rummaging through the alphabetical file to find the number, then searching for the chart itself. Because numbers were assigned consecutively as patients entered the office, the folders of members of a single family were filed all over the room. When Mrs. Jones asked, "While I'm here, would you mind checking the immunization records of my four children?" it took 15 minutes to locate the four charts. Not so, of course, when an alphabetical stystem is used. (A clever suffix scheme like the Dewey decimal system might bring the family together again, but I could never figure out a workable one.) A misplaced file card was a disaster—the patient's phantom number lost forever, his folder hidden somewhere in the stacks of numbered records. Finally, the biggest disadvantage of all was that person after person commented, "Doctor, I feel like a number, not a patient." I learned my lesson. When organizing my new office in 1968, I retreated to good old-fashioned alphabetical filing.

Microfilmed records are useful when lack of space is an acute problem, since they offer permanence and require a small fraction of the area needed to house written records. Of course, if you don't have room for a few open files along a wall, maybe you need a new office. I've resisted microfilm, having found a perfect medium for compiling records—light, portable, easily retrievable, and instantly legible without a projector. It's called paper.

All things considered, open-stack alphabetical filing of individual patient folders is the recommended method. Here are a few tips about open-stack filing: Spacers are a must, bookends and wood blocks won't do; don't economize by buying open stacks without spacers; they are needed every 6 inches. Buy open stacks at least six shelves high. Use the hard-to-reach top and bottom shelves for supply storage, until these areas are needed for filing. A sorting tray at waist level, available as an option in top-quality shelving, speeds refiling.

Planning to fill two or three side-by-side open-stack files? Place the first section of the alphabet in the first file, the second in the next, and so forth, filling only the easiest-to-reach middle shelves. Thus, you've left expansion space in the first, second, and third parts of the alphabet. If you file alphabetically straight across all our shelves, expansion involves moving every single chart.

Review your folders annually. A lot of unnecessary material can accumulate in a few years. Use a less accessible area for your inactive file. (I wish my staff would quit calling this the "dead file.") Here are stored records of patients who have died, moved away, transferred to other physicians, or failed to visit the office for at least 3 years. But don't bury that inactive file too deeply. The day you retire Mrs. Brown's chart to inactivity, she is sure to call for an appointment.

Keep your records forever. Storage space is cheap. Really it is. Don't yield to the temptation to destroy 10- and 20-year-old records. The statute of limitations on professional liability begins when a child reaches age 21. Yes, doctor, that child you delivered by breech presentation last evening, the one that had an Apgar rating of 4, may find his way to a plaintiff's attorney 23 years from now. Without your records, you're out of luck.

RECORDS THAT LEAVE YOUR OFFICE

Patients move away and are replaced by new arrivals in town. With distressing frequency, the patient's previous physician in a distant area answers my standard record-request form by shipping the complete original medical file—folder, clinical notes, and all. A letter or photocopy of the records would suffice. Never, never give or lend your original clinical records. Use your photocopier or typewriter, but keep the original records safe in your office forever.

The prudent physician reviews all photocopied records before mailing. However clever it seemed at the time, a caustic clinical note may be viewed unsympathetically by a distant doctor and your ex-patient.

X-rays and electrocardiograms are often requested by insurance companies, Workmen's Compensation carriers, and specialist-consultants. Neither photocopy well, and the examining physician should be afforded the original tracing or film. Remove the item from your file folder and note on the folder, "Loaned this date to Dr. John Smith of the XYZ Insurance Company." Then dispatch in a mailing envelope, with your specific request for its prompt return.

Industries often require preemployment physical examination of an

ROBERT B. TAYLOR, M.D.
66 FOREST GLEN ROAD
NEW PALTZ, NEW YORK 12561

AREA CODE 914
TELEPHONE 255-5450

NAME _____   DATE OF BIRTH: _____

EXAMINED FOR_____   DATE OF EXAMINATION: _____

History

Have you ever had or been treated for:

Diabetes:
Tuberculosis:
Heart Disease:
High Blood Pressure:
Back Strain:
Sciatica:
Serious injury:
Alcoholism:
Hernia:
Nervous breakdown:
Ulcer or stomach trouble:
Major Surgery:
Any Illness or Injury Not Mentioned
                    Above:

Have you ever received compensation,
    disability or other benefits due
    to illness or injury?

DETAILS:

Physical Examination

BP_____   Height_____ in.
P_____   Weight_____ lb.

Vision:
Rt. Eye: 20/   corrects to 20/
Lt. Eye: 20/   corrects to 20/

	Normal	Abnormal
Eyes:	_____	_____
Ears:	_____	_____
Oral:	_____	_____
Neck:	_____	_____
Chest:	_____	_____
Heart:	_____	_____
Abdomen	_____	_____
Back:	_____	_____
Extremities	_____	_____

Chest x-ray _____
Urine: Sugar_____; protein_____
            Microscopic:_____
Hemoglobin:_____grams

SUMMARY:

_____ Good health: recommended
                for employment

_____ Physical abnormalities as
                noted:

_____   _____
Signature of Patient   Robert B. Taylor, M.D.

Fig. 19–4. Preemployment physical examination form.

applicant, specifically requesting a detailed report. Dictate a two-page letter if you please, but why not prepare a simplified, but business-like form that you can complete while the examination is in progress. The form used in my office (Fig. 19–4) includes historical data important to employers, the patient's signature approving the history, quick check-mark notations of normal findings, a specific recommendation concerning the applicant's suitability for employment, and the physician's signature.

The computer age has added a new problem in medical records—the unsolicited computerized medical report, not infrequently concerning a person unknown to you and bearing the ominous warning, "This is the one and only copy." The problem has been dropped on your desk. If no professional relation exists between the patient and you, and you decline to accept responsibility for the report, inform the diagnostic center in writing. Return the unsolicited report with your letter via certified mail, return receipt requested, and send a copy of the letter to the patient.

If the report describes one of your patients and contains some questionable data, inform your patient in writing that a report has been received showing results that indicate further study is needed. Recommend an appointment at the patient's earliest convenience. If there has been no response within 1 week, follow-up with a certified letter, return receipt requested.

A nuisance? You bet it is? But give the matter a little thought. Is your patient visiting the "diagnostic center" because you're too busy to perform a thorough examination, or is he ignorant of your facilities? When he suffers sudden chest pain at 3 A.M. wouldn't you rather have the all-important electrocardiographic comparison tracing in your file rather than at the diagnostic center, safely locked up for the night?

References and Suggestions for Further Reading

1. Bjorn J C, Cross H D: Problem-oriented Practice. New York, McGraw-Hill, 1970.
2. Bjorn J C, Cross H D: The Problem-Oriented Private Practice of Medicine: A System for Comprehensive Health Care. Chicago, Modern Hospital Press, 1970.
3. Bourke G J, McGilvray J: Interpretation and Uses of Medical Statistics. Philadelphia, Davis, 1969.
4. Chamberlin R W Jr: Social data in evaluation of the pediatric patient: Deficits in outpatient records. J Pediatr 78:111–116, 1971.
5. Dixon W J, Massey F J: Introduction to Statistical Analysis. New York, McGraw-Hill, 1957.
6. Enslein K: Conference on Data Acquisition and Processing in Biology and Medicine. Elmsford, NY, Pergamon, 1968.

7. Fox R M: The Medical Report: Theory and Practice. Boston, Little, Brown, 1969.

8. Hurst J W: How to implement the Weed system. Arch Intern Med 128:456–462, 1971.

9. Hurst J W: Ten reasons why Lawrence Weed is right. N Engl J Med 284:51–52, 1971.

10. Norden A: Research in general practice. World Med J 18:14–17, 1971.

11. Oldham P D: Measurement in Medicine. Philadelphia, Lippincott, 1968.

12. Schulman J, Wood C: Flow sheets for charts of ambulatory patients. JAMA 217:-933–937, 1971.

13. Vawter S M, Deforest R E: The international metric system and medicine. JAMA 218:723–726, 1971.

20

The Light Side of Office Practice

Health and cheerfulness mutually beget each other.

Joseph Addison
(1672–1719)

Sick and healthy patients alike crave cheerful surroundings, a smiling face, and a pleasant voice. Who wants to visit an office with the odor of an operating theater, the darkness of a dungeon, and gloom of a mortuary? There's no reason why the doctor's office can't be as inviting as the local shoe store or beauty parlor.

As retail businesses learned decades ago, it's the "little extras" that bring customers (or patients) back. A smiling nurse's praise of the patient's 3-lb weight loss can be a valuable stimulus, and the promise of a token gift can dissolve a 4-year-old's aversion to doctors. Most extras take more imagination than money, but return the priceless dividend of grateful patients.

HAPPINESS IS A CHEERFUL PATIENT

Your aide's first duty is to be cheerful; machines can record accounts and answer the telephone. Maybe she can't always give the appointment wanted or get the insurance form completed today, but she can do it cheerfully. If garish hamburger palaces can train high-school dropouts to exude competence and good humor, your employees can learn too.

Your patient's visit begins in the waiting room, although hopefully he remains there only long enough to complete an insurance form or skim a brief magazine article. (Chapter 21 tells how to eliminate endless waiting-room incarcerations.) Brighten your patient's day by providing up-to-date issues of unusual magazines, such as *Saturday Review, Travel,* or *Ski,* in addition to *Life, Time,* and *Newsweek.* Don't neglect the youngsters. *Highlights for Children* and *Children's Digest* are always welcomed by smallfry. Don't forget that historical standby of waiting rooms through the ages, *National Geographic.* But please keep your *Medical Economics* and *Physician's Management* in your consultation room; candid articles about fees and professional liability aren't intended for your waiting room.

A writing desk in the waiting room speeds completion of insurance forms. Stock the stationery drawer with blank health plan forms so the patient need not wait his turn at the front desk. If the only writing surface in the waiting room is your checkout counter, form completion can monopolize the front desk. The writing table frees you aide's checkout area for more important matters. The children's area of the waiting room frees armchairs for adults and keeps children where you want them—away from walls and table lamps. A sturdy child's play table with matching chairs can conveniently be placed in the middle of the waiting room, allowing mothers to keep an eye on their offspring. Leave a few children's periodicals on the play table. I stock my children's area with small coloring books and crayons.

Bulletin boards can be fun. Every waiting room needs at least one, bearing immunization reminders and items of current medical interest to patients. How about a poster board displaying your pediatric patients' artistic efforts with crayons and coloring book? My hometown dentist displayed a gaily decorated poster titled, "The I-Can-Take-It-Club," where proud young patients were allowed to sign up upon completion of treatment. Dr. Herbert Weinman of New Paltz, New York, sports a baby picture board, exhibiting candid Polaroid snapshots of his pediatric patients and affording a pictorial record of the babies' development.

Seasonal decorations brighten holiday seasons. A miniature Christmas tree with unbreakable wooden ornaments can be stored from year to year. Halloween, Easter, and Valentine's Day decorations can be made by pediatric patients or perhaps your own children. And don't forget to display the American flag on Memorial Day, Veterans' Day, and the Fourth of July.

A local artist or art association might welcome the opportunity to exhibit paintings in your waiting room. Have plenty of wall space? Invite a revolving exhibit, featuring different local artists, changed at monthly intervals.

PATIENT PLEASERS

A white coat commands respect and conveys an aura of clinical austerity. It also frightens the blazes out of youngsters. In the office, a colored short-sleeved shirt is less terrifying to toddlers and allows greater freedom of movement.

Patients gag watching you extract a lint covered tongue blade from your pocket. "Is he going to put that unsterile thing in my mouth?" He may not verbalize it, but your patient appreciates individually wrapped tongue blades, the covering removed to reveal a hospital-sterile, lint-free tongue depressor.

Examination-room waits can seem interminable. Separated from his family, isolated in a stark cubicle, the patient awaits the doctor's arrival. Adults stare out the window and worry. Children play with your instruments. Give them something to do: Allow youngsters to bring a waiting-room magazine or coloring book with them. Adults can tote a magazine. If long waits are the rule, leave a few periodicals in the examination room. I use a pamphlet rack, containing timely health bulletins available at no cost from your local Heart Association, Cancer Society, Mental Health Clinic, pharmaceutical companies (Ross Laboratories, P.O. Box 688, Columbus, Ohio, 43216, has excellent pamphlets), or the Metropolitan Life Insurance Company. Free to take home after the visit, pamphlets ease the frantic fidgets.

Gowning female patients can be awkward. The full-length examination gown or sheet is acceptable for inspection of the chest or pelvis; but the abdominal examination poses problems, embarrassingly exposing top or bottom. Some clinics use a silly little towel for modesty. The best solution is two-piece gowning (Fig. 20–1), using a short gown and a half-sheet, preserving dignity and facilitating examination of the abdomen. Color-code by using green sheet material for the short gown and another color for the bottom half-sheet, to eliminate unfolding to find the one you want. A local seamstress can copy commercial patterns, using the new permanent press fabrics. Avoid nylon or rayon; slippery fabrics slide off patients.

Your aide gowns the ladies and remains in the room as chaperone during the examination. Big-city doctors tell of attractive young addicts who disrobe in the examination room, smile, and threaten, "Doctor, give me $50 or I'll scream!" It could happen to you. A silent buzzer to summon your aide helps, but a chaperone in the room is better.

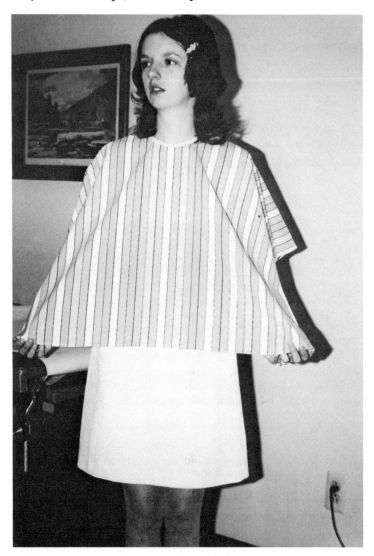

Fig. 20–1. Two-piece gown for female patients.

Some patients can't lie flat—suffering from rheumatoid spondylitis, congestive heart failure, or dowager's hump. Raising the table still does not support the head, and tight abdominal muscles thwart examination. My nurse suggested a round bolster pillow behind the neck to support the head and relax the rectus abdominis.

Mirrors add depth to cramped examination rooms and amuse children. Ladies can adjust their make-up and men their ties. A hand mirror lets your patient see his new facial sutures. The lavatories, examination rooms, and treatment room should all contain mirrors.

Many a crisis is averted by stocking a few simple items. Consider these before the need arises:

1. Disposable diapers for the infant who has just soaked his last one
2. Sanitary pads for the woman with vaginal bleeding
3. Ready-to-use infant formula samples for the hungry baby detained past mealtime
4. A wooden cane to assist sprained ankle victims on their trip home (use a wood burner to inscribe your name on the shaft)
5. A loan umbrella, for that sudden deluge (again identify with a name tag)
6. Safety pins for emergency treatment of broken zippers or repair of trousers split to accommodate a cast

In most areas of the country, the dispensing doctor departed with high-buttoned shoes and horse-drawn buggies. The corner pharmacy boasts a larger stock than any doctor's office should contain; but think about it. Are there three or four prescriptions you write over and over? Penicillin tablets? Tetracycline capsules? Prednisone tablets? Throat lozenges? It won't increase your income, but consider stocking these low-cost generic medications, prepackaged in the usual dosage, and dispensed as "part of the office visit." (Selling medication puts you in the drug store business and exposes you to possible governmental disapproval.) Twenty penicillin-G tablets cost the physician about 35 cents. Dispensed in clear plastic vials with preprinted labels bearing your name, address, telephone number, the patient's name, and date can spare your patient's pocketbook and earn his gratitude.

A cuddly stuffed animal may comfort a crying 2-year-old. We have Oscar, a threadbare monkey, left unclaimed in the waiting room several years ago. Oscar, the orphan, has been adopted by dozens of local children; many ask for him upon arrival, care for him during their visit, and surrender the toy upon departing.

Give-away toys reduce a child's natural reluctance to visit the doctor and dry tears after an injection. The average preschooler is a greedy little rascal. He can't produce a urine specimen or cooperate with audiometry? Promise a toy as a reward and see how he responds. My office stocks brightly colored novelty rings for older youngsters and plastic cars (that can't be swallowed) for toddlers. Probably available from a local medical, dental, or novelty supply dealer, my source is the Mapac Company, Bellmore, New York. Avoid lollipop prizes; your dental colleagues will frown.

WHAT DID THE DOCTOR SAY? NOTHING

Did you ever listen to waiting-room conversation? John Patient leaves your consultation room, following a learned exposition concerning the response of the gastric mucosa to emotional tension and dietary indiscretion. Out to the waiting room he bounds. His wife looks up expectantly, "What did the doctor say you have, John?" "Nothing. It's all in my mind."

Patients leave a medical consultation retaining only about a quarter of what you said. But they study drawings, follow diets, read handouts, and obey written instructions. Whenever possible, supplement your explanations with documentation.

Pogo once said: "Words are for people who can't read pictures." A simple line drawing demonstrates how low back strain occurs or unlocks the mysteries of eustachian tube blockage. Keep a scratch pad handy and draw as you talk; you'll be surprised how many drawings are taken home along with your prescriptions.

Demonstration charts help. Most pharmaceutical companies offer helpful laminated drawings that expedite explanations by illustrating the inner workings of the heart, stomach, and joints. For example, the Smith, Kline & French Laboratories, Philadelphia, Pennsylvania, offer physicians multiple plastic drawings of various organs with tissue-paper overlays for easy demonstration of pathology.

Plastic models demonstrate joint function. Some move and others come apart to reveal the inner workings of tendons, ligaments, arteries, and joint cavities. An excellent series of models has been distributed by Geigy Pharmaceuticals, Ardsley, New York.

Printed instructions and diets supplement consultation and give the patient tangible evidence of therapy. A few evenings at the typewriter can produce personalized instructions, incorporating your own imaginative therapeutic techniques. An example is the acute ulcer diet shown in Figure 20–2, developed to guide patients through the first days of peptic ulcer or gastritis therapy. Typed on your letterhead, personalized instructions are easily reproduced by your local printer. Even handwritten or ineptly typed material can be salvaged by instructing the printer to set type. Lack the literary bent to compose your own instructions? Then purchase H. Winter Griffith's *Instructions for Patients*, a comprehensive loose-leaf folder offering explanations, diets, and treatment regimens—intended for duplication on your office photocopier.

ROBERT B. TAYLOR, M.D.
66 FOREST GLEN ROAD
NEW PALTZ, NEW YORK 12561

AREA CODE 914
TELEPHONE 255-5450

ACUTE PEPTIC ULCER DIET

General Diet Rules

NO FOOD TO BE EATEN EXCEPT AS SHOWN BELOW. FEEDINGS MUST BE TAKEN REGULARLY AS LISTED. MILK SHOULD BE AT ROOM TEMPERATURE. NO ALCOHOLIC DRINKS.

8 A.M.	One portion of cooked Farina, Wheatena or Cream of Wheat with sugar and ½ glass of cream. One slice of toasted white bread with butter. One glass of milk.
10 A.M.	One glass of eggnog, malted milk, buttermilk or Half and Half.
12 Noon	One portion of cream soup with strained vegetables, such as celery, mushrooms, or asparagus. Mashed, baked or boiled potato with butter. Plain Jello. Cornstarch, custard, rice or tapioca pudding. Junket.
2 P.M.	One glass of milk.
4 P.M.	One glass of eggnog, malted milk, buttermilk or Half and Half.
6 P.M.	Small cup of cream soup with vegetables. Mashed, baked or boiled potato with butter. Small portion of white meat of chicken or turkey, flounder, or poached egg. One glass of milk.
8 P.M.	One glass of milk.
Bedtime	One glass of eggnog, malted milk, buttermilk or Half and Half.

Antacid medication, such as Maalox, Mylanta, or Riopan, may be taken as often as every two hours if needed for abdominal distress.

Fig. 20–2. Printed diet instructions for the patient with acute peptic ulcer.

"Did the doctor say Johnny needs a polio shot this year?" Try as they may, parents never remember when immunizations are due. Send them an immunization reminder card (Fig. 20–3). Your office nurse can put her spare time to good use by reviewing an entire family's clinical

ROBERT B. TAYLOR, M.D.
66 FOREST GLEN ROAD
NEW PALTZ, NEW YORK 12561

——

AREA CODE 914
TELEPHONE 255-5450

Date_____

Dear Mrs._____:

Many serious childhood illnesses are prevented by keeping immunizations up-to-date.
A review of our records indicates that your children need the following immunizations to keep them up-to-date:

Name_____

_____ DPT or Tetanus booster
_____ Small pox vaccination
_____ Sabin oral polio
_____ Rubella vaccine
_____ Measles vaccine (if he has not had measles)
_____ Mumps vaccine (if he has not had mumps)
_____ We do not have a complete shot record on this child. Would you please send it to us so that our records may be kept up to date.

Name_____

_____ DPT or Tetanus booster
_____ Small Pox vaccination
_____ Sabin oral polio
_____ Rubella vaccine
_____ Measles vaccine (if he has not had measles)
_____ Mumps vaccine (if he has not had mumps)
_____ We do not have a complete shot record on this child. Would you please send it to us so that our records may be kept up to date.

Name_____

_____ DPT or Tetanus booster
_____ Small Pox vaccination
_____ Sabin oral polio
_____ Rubella vaccine
_____ Measles vaccine (if he has not had measles)
_____ Mumps vaccine (if he has not had mumps)
_____ We do not have a complete shot record on this child. Would you please send it to us so that our records may be kept up to date.

You may call for an appointment for these immunizations at your convenience.

Very truly yours,

for _____Robert B. Taylor, M.D.

Fig. 20–3. Immunization-reminder form.

records and listing immunizations needed. She can check two or three letters of the alphabet each month, or if the folders are color-coded, all charts of one color each month.

"What did the doctor say?" "Oh, all we talked about was golf." We all tire of discussing coughs and constipation. Sometimes, when the patient is a social acquaintance, the doctor falls prey to the urge to chit-chat. While examining the ears, he tells about his birdie last week. While he palpates the abdomen, the sand trap on the fourth hole is condemned. Quietly the patient smolders. However witty your small talk, it's not worth the price your patient is paying for the consultation. Stick to business until the medical consultation is over. Having a slow day? Time on your hands? Really want to chat? Then conclude the consultation with, "Now have we covered everything?" If so, then lean back and relax a few minutes with your pal.

"Did the doctor find out what's wrong?" "He doesn't know what he is talking about. I'm going to see another physician." Trouble here. Somehow the doctor-patient relation has broken down, and the fault probably lies with the physician. They have a saying in business: "The customer is always right." Illness increases emotional lability, resentment that should be directed toward the malady often is heaped upon the doctor. Don't reply in kind. Try to see your patient's viewpoint and express your sincere desire to solve his problem. If he deplores the high cost of medication, remind him "What you spend for medicine in 1 year won't pay for 1 day in the hospital." To his worries about the income lost by a week out of work reply "A week of rest now may prevent a month lost later." If he's concerned over a slow response to therapy, reassure him, "There's always one patient who recovers slowly. You're the one. Let's work together to solve the problem."

In a letter to Dr. William Claypoole on July 29, 1782, Dr. Benjamin Rush wrote: "Never resent an affront offered to you by a sick man. . . . Never make light (to a patient) of any case. Never appear in a hurry in a sickroom, nor talk of indifferent matters till you have examined and prescribed for your patient."

References and Suggestions for Further Reading

1. Bates R: The Fine Art of Understanding Patients. Oradell, NJ, Medical Economics Book Division, 1968.
2. Blum R H: The Management of the Doctor-Patient Relationship. New York, McGraw-Hill, 1960.
3. Brook A, Bleasdale J K, Dowling S J: Emotional problems in general practice: A sample of ordinary patients. J Coll Gen Practice 11:184–194, 1966.

4. Browne K, Freeling P: The Doctor-Patient Relationship. Baltimore, Williams & Wilkins, 1967.

5. Griffith H W: Instructions for Patients. Philadelphia, Saunders, 1968.

6. Hollender M H: The Psychology of Medical Practice. Philadelphia, Saunders, 1958.

7. Ramsey P: The Patient as Person. New Haven, Yale University Press, 1970.

8. Robins R B: The Environment of Medical Practice. Chicago, Year Book, 1963.

9. Steiger W A, Hansen A V Jr: Patients Who Trouble You. Boston, Little, Brown, 1964.

10. Wearn J T: Cherish the capacity to change. Calif Med 106:375–381, 1967.

21

How To Get Home in Time for Dinner

Practical medicine is never the same thing as scientific medicine but rather, even in the hands of the greatest master, an application of it.

Rudolf Virchow
(1821–1902)

Yes, even the great masters, such as Benjamin Rush and Sir William Osler, outstanding physicians who have earned their niches in medical history, were faced by the day-to-day problem of getting patients in and out of the office, hopefully completing office hours in time for dinner and a few quiet hours with the family. Practice productivity isn't measured by hours spent in the office, but by patients properly treated per working hour. An inefficient physician, dawdling until 11 P.M. each evening, is less valuable to his patients than his well-organized colleague who handles problems with dispatch, ends his day at a reasonable hour, and is rested to face evening emergencies.

A smooth running practice is like a finely tuned engine—operating at peak efficiency without strain. Lubricate your creaky methods to smooth the flow of patients.

APPOINTMENT SYSTEMS

Have you ever seen mothers who, weary of restraining restless children after 90 minutes in the waiting room, turn the kids loose, hoping that the ensuing melee will bring her family to the doctor's attention? A 90-minute wait is a symptom of a sick appointment system. So are telephone calls inquiring, "I have an appointment in 10 minutes. How long will I have to wait?" Is your office renowned for long waits, hoards of patients stacked side-by-side in the waiting room? Then pay attention and take action in your practice.

An appointment system can only speed your day. The longer a patient sits in the waiting room, the more time he expects to spend with the doctor. Whether your patients read the *National Geographic* for 2 hours or 10 minutes, you can treat at least as many patients by appointment as without; and you can prevent that worried face peering in the door to see, "How many are ahead of me," viewing the mob, and deciding to go elsewhere. That's fine for a barber shop, but not a medical office.

There are really three appointment systems: the pool, the wave, and the stream. Review them carefully and pick the one that's right for you.

The pool system is really no system at all. A placard on Dr. Brown's office door announces: "Office hours from 1 to 5 P.M." By noon the queue has begun to form, sick and well alike, waiting for the show to begin. The door is unlocked and in they dash, scrambling for the best seats, anticipating a good long wait. Enter the doctor. With 10 or 15 patients squirming expectantly, he is already 2 hours behind. On he plods through the afternoon, dismal at the prospect of the 4:45 onslaught, when the after-work and after-school mob strikes. After all, his sign implies that all arrivals before 5 P.M. will be treated. Will he get home in time for dinner? Not a chance, unless the dinner hour is 10 P.M.

The wave system is used in many large clinics and has some advantages. But like the pool system, it can unnecessarily prolong waiting-room time. In the wave system, three to five appointments are scheduled hourly. As the clock chimes, the 10 A.M. or 11 A.M. throng arrives and the patients are treated on a first-come basis. The advantages? No-shows and late arrivals don't disrupt your schedule. The wave system assumes that brief visits will balance prolonged ones and minimizes the questioning needed to scheduling appointments appropriately. Theoretically, each hour ends with a catch-up period before the next wave strikes. Disadvantages? The catch-up period, if it occurs at all, is really wasted time. And patients talk, "Do you have a 2 o'clock appointment? So do I!" "I do, too," chime in other voices. Not very good patient relations.

The stream system flows patients through the office smoothly, but takes effort and careful aide training. A suture removal consumes less time than an earache, which, in turn, requires fewer minutes than a complete physical examination. A smooth-flowing stream appointment system requires a capable aide who carefully questions each patient concerning the nature of his visit. Before long, she gets a feeling for the correct time allotment. When functioning properly, the stream system eliminates idle minutes and restless patients.

How about emergencies? Do they wreck your schedule? Most general offices begin the day with few truly open appointments that are filled rapidly in the morning. Then emergencies and call-ins must be accommodated. Be rigid here or the day's end will be a disaster. Sure, almost all your call-ins would like to come at 4:30, after school or when Daddy comes home from work. Efficient call-in scheduling dictates that urgent appointments are filled from the top down. You're extending yourself to squeeze the patient in that day. Be firm about the time offered or you'll be facing a huge sickly mob at quitting time.

Your appointment book can be purchased commercially or printed to your specifications (it really isn't expensive). For a single-doctor office, the appointment log should have three columns (Fig. 21–1). The first column contains routine appointments, filled in careful stream fashion before the second column is started. The second column is for call-in appointments, two per hour, filled *consecutively* beginning in the morning. Call-in appointments are just that, and column 2 should remain virgin until the day begins. The third column contains nurse's appointments for patients who need not see the doctor (routine immunizations, physical therapy, and laboratory tests).

Here are a few extra scheduling tips: If you find that your first patient of the morning or afternoon is always late, leaving you nervously pacing, double-schedule these appointments to get you going. Do you find that your end-of-the-day appointments often arrive late? Then schedule your 4, 4:15, and 4:30 P.M. patients all for 4 o'clock—a small concession to the wave system that will prevent that interminable wait for the last patient to arrive.

The return appointment slip (Fig. 21–2) tells your aide when the patient should return, how much time will be needed, what preparation the patient should make (fasting, enema, laxative), and what procedures are planned (x-ray, cast removal, or sigmoidoscopy).

Whatever your system, the girl on the telephone must find out what the patient has in mind. Some patients are better sent to the hospital

	DOCTOR'S APPOINTMENTS	EMERGENCIES CALL-INS	NURSE'S APPOINTMENTS
8:30		1.	
45			
9:00	Complete	2.	
15	Physical		
30	Examination	3.	
45	-------		
10:00		4.	
15			
30		5.	
45			
11:00		6.	
15			
30		7.	
45			
12:00	-------	-------	-------
15	-------	-------	-------
30	-------	-------	-------
45	-------	-------	-------
1:00		8.	
15			
30		9.	
45			
2:00		10.	
15			
30		11.	
45			
3:00		12.	
15			
30		13.	
45			
4:00		14.	
15			
30		15.	
45			
5:00			

Fig. 21–1. Appointment scheduling for the solo office.

```
Robert B. Taylor, M.D.
66 Forest Glen Rd.
New Paltz, N.Y., 12561

RETURN APPOINTMENT SLIP

Patient_____

Should return in
     (exactly, approximately):

     _____ days

     _____ weeks

     _____ months

To see:

     _____ Dr. Taylor

     _____ Nurse

Allow _____minutes for the visit.

For the visit the patient should:

_____

At the visit, we plan to:

_____
```

Fig. 21–2. Return appointment slip.

(hip fractures or extensive lacerations), and some require more time than you have available that day. The patient who "wants the doctor to look at a mole" very likely wants it removed. Removal takes more time than looking. Schedule accordingly. Have you ever been faced with a squeezed-in (emergency) patient who announces, "Well, Doctor, I'm here for my complete physical examination"? Then you understand why intelligent aides are important.

Patients cancel and reschedule appointments, often on short notice, leaving huge gaps in your schedule unless there's a second stringer to send in. Your aide should note patients who wanted routine appointments but were met with crowded schedules and forced to accept times next week. When a long appointment is canceled on a day's notice or less, call in the other waiting patient.

Should you charge for missed appointments? When an appointment is not kept, my office calls the patient, reminding him that his appointment was important to us as well as to him. Car broke down on the road? An emergency at home? Couldn't call? Then forget it (the first time at least). But if the patient just changed his mind, decided to do something else, or thought it wasn't important, a token charge (let's say $5) is a forceful deterrent to repeat performances.

HOW TO SEE MORE PATIENTS IN LESS TIME

With rising overhead, oppressive fee ceilings, and rising taxes, the struggling physician can maintain financial solvency only through increased practice productivity—more patients seen each hour. The luxuries of the leisurely office visit and convenience house call are gone forever.

House calls gobble time, particularly annoying when the justification for a home visit is a lack of transportation or the mother's insistence that, "I don't want Johnny to go outdoors with his cold." Certainly it would be gratifying to treat all respiratory infections at home, but a busy doctor can care for eight office patients while making two house calls. Simply stated, almost all sick patients must be treated in the office; house calls are reserved for those truly too sick to be moved.

But the pressures of time are your problem, not Mrs. Jones'. Her sole concern is her sick child. Somehow, tactfully, your aide must convince Mrs. Jones that it is to *her* advantage to bring Johnny in. Here's the way it's done: "Mrs. Jones, the Doctor's appointments are completely filled all day and he couldn't get to your home until after dinner. You could save Johnny several hours by bringing him to the office now. Warm up the car and come to the emergency entrance. We'll be looking for you and take him right in without waiting." It usually works, to everyone's satisfaction as long as you keep your no-waiting promise.

Increased practice productivity means getting the most out of every minute. Time spent watching an elderly patient struggle with his coat and tie represents productive minutes wasted. As the aide admits your patient to the examination room, she should anticipate your needs, instructing youngsters to remove their sweaters and older patients their outer garments.

Three-session visits slow the office pace. Usually involving female patients, session 1 yields the history, session 2 involves the physical examination, and session 3 the final consultation. What a waste of time! A clever aide could anticipate that Mrs. Smith's cough and fever will entail a chest examination. With the patient already gowned, a potential three-session office call is concluded in one brief episode.

The *Physician's Desk Reference (PDR)* is an invaluable aid in finding drug dosage and identifying unknown tablets. Need you go to your consultation room library each time you want to check a drug dosage? Not if each examination room contains its own *PDR*. The *PDR* is updated and mailed to physicians annually by Medical Economics, Inc., Oradell, New Jersey. Additional copies are available at a modest price, but with yearly additions rolling in, your office soon contains four or five volumes from past years, allowing placement of an issue in each examination room.

It takes more time to care for healthy people than sick ones. School physical examinations can be particularly time-consuming, especially if you perform a thorough check-up, as I do, including urine analysis, visual acuity, audiometry, and an exhaustive physical examination. After all that, there are forms to fill in. My office can survive the simultaneous visits of two siblings for school examinations, but the third brother or sister slows the wheels—too many immunization records, audiograms, and forms. A single examination room is tied up for more than 30 minutes—too long in a busy practice. And if the mother has to cancel, erasing three or four back-to-back appointments leaves a gaping wound in the day's schedule. The moral of the story? No more than two school physicals in any family on any given day.

The secret of successful office practice today is rushing without appearing rushed. You may feel you're running on a treadmill, but your patient should leave the office convinced that he has just concluded a leisurely unhurried consultation. The secret? Stick to the subject. Choose your words carefully and avoid darting off on tangents. Summarize your advice, then rise indicating the completion of the interview. Save your chit-chat for the country club. There are still patients waiting to be seen.

NURSING DUTIES ARE FOR NURSES

The modern nurse is well trained in the theory and practice of hospital medicine. Most know precious little about office medical care and have never performed an electrocardiogram, operated an audiometer, determined visual acuity, or administered an ultrasound treatment. Yes, some postgraduate training is necessary, with tutoring by the head nurse or the doctor himself. The breaking in of a new aide is an excellent opportunity to begin good habits that will save the office time and money.

Why have aides? The doctor pays good money for assistants to free his time for demanding professional duties. In an efficient office, an aide performs every function not requiring professional judgment and an M.D. degree. That's her job—seeing that the physician spends his time doctoring, not weighing patients, making appointments, or completing insurance forms.

What is the nurse's first priority? Keep the doctor busy! The office moves as fast or slow as the doctor. Break his stride with empty rooms and dawdling patients, and watch the waiting-room mob grow. When your aide has to decide between administering an injection and preparing a patient for the doctor, there's only one choice: Keep the doctor busy.

In the quest for perpetual busyness, the doctor should issue standing orders to his staff:

1. Give all patients a charge slip and record fees when a service is performed

2. Weigh all patients who have not been examined for 3 months or more

3. Weigh and measure all infants and children receiving routine physical examinations; figure and record percentiles

4. Obtain urine for analysis from all patients receiving routine physical examinations or complaining of abdominal pain, back pain, or difficulty with urination

5. Record the temperature of all patients with acute illness, whether complaining of fever or not

6. Perform visual acuity tests on all patients with eye complaints

7. Perform audiometry on all patients with ear symptoms

8. Have mothers begin disrobing children before the doctor enters

9. Keep the flow of patients moving

Rewriting known prescriptions is an exercise in penmanship, requiring only the physician's review and signature. Teach your nurses to write prescriptions; usually the local pharmacist will be glad to dictate the prescription when renewal time comes around. Careful charting allows your nurse to copy prescriptions from the record, and those pesky "no refill" union and welfare fund prescriptions can become her bailiwick. But, always and forever, retain the prerogative of final review and signature.

When do I find time to teach all my aides (I have two full-time and seven part-time aides) all these procedures? Day-by-day training helps. But when a new procedure is introduced or some minor techniques require updating, we hold a staff meeting. Scheduled during lunch on a day that doesn't look too busy, the staff meeting allows a one-time explanation of new and old problems. Everyone attends. Luncheon is catered (hot sandwiches). The open discussion of office policies and the feeling of camaraderie engendered by luncheon staff meetings certainly justify the small expense and brief loss of office working time.

TIME WASTERS

Mr. Parkinson said it: "Duties will expand to exceed the time allotted to them." The path to patient productivity is full of perils with sirens to entice you into time-wasting habits. Fill your ears with wax to drown the sweet song of idleness and lash yourself to the mast of self-discipline.

Take the coffee lounge in the hospital surgical suite, for instance. How many valuable man-hours are wasted here daily? Get in and out of the hospital early—as early as 7 or 7:30 A.M.—missing the parking lot traffic jam, the competition for nurses' attention, and the temptation to chat with your colleagues.

Has a colleague (or even you) ever declined a case because of a committee meeting? What a paradox? Patient care going begging while doctors meet to discuss patient care. Certainly, hospitals need committees—at least they and federal inspectors think so. But avoid committee entanglements. Shun chairmanship as though it were *T. pallidum* himself. Serve on your obligatory one committee yearly, avoid distinction, and never volunteer. Your patients are more important that committees.

Are some days consumed by transcribing Medicaid prescriptions? Why do all Medicaid patients seem to take six medications regularly? And, just think, when Congress, in its all-knowing wisdom, passes the cost of Medicare prescriptions on to the taxpayers, all senior citizens will require monthly prescription rewriting. Your aide can copy the prescriptions if they can all be located easily. Try the prescription renewal form (Fig. 21–3). If your local social service agency will allow it, the doctor need only check the medications to refill, date and sign the form. Does the Welfare Department insist upon its own forms? Then your aide can easily copy the data, once the prescription renewal form is in hand. You need only date and sign your name.

In almost all cases, request that the pharmacist identify medication on the package label. It can save valuable minutes—time otherwise spent thumbing through the *PDR*.

Finley Peter Dunn (Mr. Dooley) (1867–1936) wrote: "I wondher why

ROBERT B. TAYLOR, M.D.
66 FOREST GLEN ROAD
NEW PALTZ, NEW YORK 12561

TELEPHONE 914-255-5450

PRESCRIPTION RENEWAL

If you want a repeat prescription, this form
should be brought to the office a few days before
your medication runs out. Hand this form to the
nurse and tell her which medications need refills.
No appointment is needed. Telephone requests for
repeat prescriptions cannot be accepted.

Name: _____   Telephone: _____

Address: _____   Date of Birth: _____

_____

MEDICATIONS

Name of Drug	Dose	Disp. No.	Directions	Number of Refills	Fill Only Rx Checked
___	___	___	___	___	___
___	___	___	___	___	___
___	___	___	___	___	___
___	___	___	___	___	___
___	___	___	___	___	___
___	___	___	___	___	___
___	___	___	___	___	___

Please Note Name of Medication
on Package Label

BNDD No. 1234567   Signature: _____

Date Authorized: _____

Fig. 21–3. Prescription renewal form.

ye can always read a doctor's bill an' ye niver can read his purscription."
But the patient can always spell the identifying package label, facilitating conversation when he telephones to inquire about medication.

Scheduling x-rays at the hospital (upper gastrointestinal series, cholecystography, intravenous pyelography) takes time. But it should be your aide's time, not yours. Here's a hint to speed the process: Prepare a preprinted form, listing the recommended preparation for common x-rays (Fig. 21–4). Once the examination is scheduled, check the appropriate paragraph and hand the form to your patient. Without a standard x-ray preparation form, your secretary must type new directions each time.

Waiting for an open telephone line can make your ulcer bleed (your secretary has a patient on one line while she makes an appointment on another). Sure, your call may not be urgent, but waiting wastes minutes. Do you have enough telephone lines? Are patients repeatedly getting busy signals, unknown to you? Find out by asking the telephone company to run a "busy check" for a few days, pinpointing the number of calls resulting in that annoying busy buzz-buzz-buzz.

If your telephone lines hum, and outgoing calls present a problem, install a "hot line" in your consultation room. The number should be unlisted, known only to your family, staff, and professional associates. When the front desk telephone lights are all lit, the "hot line" is open for your call.

Some senior citizens come for two purposes: a medical consultation, followed by a prolonged discussion of Medicare benefits, involving those maddening computer printouts from the regional Medicare intermediary. Stop the discussion. "My secretary handles all Medicare inquiries. She deals with these problems daily and has more experience than I. Please review your forms with her, and we'll do everything we can to help." Much as you would like to be helpful, your time is too valuable to be spent explaining insurance benefits.

HOW TO END AN INTERVIEW

Some patients love to chat. Heedless of the time, they drone on, detailing the trivia that crowds their waking hours. Someone, somewhere, told these patients, "Always tell your doctor everything." They will.

When the medical history becomes repetitious and endless, wait for the patient to draw a breath; then say, "Okay. Let's find out what's wrong. Take off your shirt (or the nurse will gown you), and let's get on with the examination." This ploy works. The physical examination is really why the patient came to you. He could have detailed his history in a letter.

He's still talking during the examination? Then tell him to breathe

ROBERT B. TAYLOR, M.D.
66 FOREST GLEN ROAD
NEW PALTZ, NEW YORK 12561

———

AREA CODE 914
TELEPHONE 255-5450

<u>PREPARATION FOR X-RAY EXAMINATIONS</u>

FOLLOW <u>ONLY</u> THE DIRECTIONS CHECKED:

___ <u>GALLBLADDER</u>:

No fatty food at evening meal.

Take 6 Telepaque tablets between 9 and 11 the
night before, one at a time.

May have "gallbladder" breakfast. No fatty
foods (dry toast, tea, or coffee without
milk). Omit breakfast if x-rays include
upper G.I. series.

___ <u>UPPER GI SERIES</u>:

Nothing to eat or drink from midnight on.

___ <u>BARIUM ENEMA</u>:

1 ounce of Castor oil or 1½ ounces of Fleets
Phosphosoda at 4 p.m. (day before examination).

___ <u>IVP</u>

1 ounce of Fleets Phosphosoda taken at 4 p.m.
day before examination.

Regular evening meal.

Nothing to eat or drink after evening meal.

Report to the_____Hospital X-ray

Department at _(time)_ a.m./p.m. on__(date)__.

Fig. 21–4. Form explaining preparation needed for x-ray examination.

slowly, in and out, through his mouth. Let's see him keep talking while doing that. Of course, give him a rest every few minutes lest hyperventilation lead to syncope.

The history and physical examination completed, the garrulous patient continues talking. Here's how to end the visit: When your host becomes repetitive, it's time to leave the party. Begin repeating the advice you have already given. Summarize your recommendations, assure the patient that he should feel better soon, hand him the charge slip, stand up, shake his hand, open the door, and smile, "I've certainly enjoyed talking with you. I could chat all day, but I'm afraid I have to get back to work."

References and Suggestions for Further Reading

1. Bevan J, Draper G J: Appointment Systems in General Practice. New York, Oxford University Press, 1967.
2. Bird B: Talking with Patients. Philadelphia, Lippincott, 1955.
3. Bogdonoff M D: Concern about patient care. Arch Intern Med 123:719–721, 1969.
4. Clyne M G: Night Calls: A Study in General Practice. Philadelphia, Lippincott, 1961.
5. Coye R D, Hansen M F: The "doctor's assistant." JAMA 209:529–533, 1969.
6. Froelich R E, Bishop M: Medical Interviewing: A Programmed Manual. St Louis, Mosby, 1969.
7. Gonella J A, Goran M J, Williamson J W: The evaluation of patient care: A new approach. JAMA 214:2040–2043, 1970.
8. Griffith H W: Instructions for Patients. Philadelphia, Saunders, 1968.
9. Kimball C P: Interviewing, diagnosis and therapy. Postgrad Med 47:88–93, 1970.
10. Nithman C J, Parkhurst Y E, Sommers E B: Physicians' prescribing habits. JAMA 217:585–587, 1971.
11. Smith R A, Bassett G R, Markarian C A, Vath R E, Freeman W L, Dunn G F: A strategy for health manpower. JAMA 217:1362–1367, 1971.
12. Stevenson I: The Diagnostic Interview. New York, Harper & Row, 1971.
13. Taylor R B: This prescription form saves time. Physician's Management 12:3 p.78–0–79–0, 1972.

22

Those Pesky Third Parties

The well-equipped clinician must possess the qualities of the artist, the man of science, and the humanist, but he must exercise them only in so far as they subserve the getting well of the individual patient. He must feel directly responsible to his patient, not for him —to someone else.

Sir Alfred Webb-Johnson
(1880–1958)

Perhaps in the twenty-first century, medical schools will offer a course in the interpretation and completion of insurance forms. Sad to say, medical practice has already reached the era when creative responses to insurance forms can augment the doctor's income faster than any amount of increased training and experience.

Who pay your bills, doctor? Who do you really work for? I'll tell you. You work for the man who pays you. If you submit your statement to the insurance company, beseechingly grateful for the pittance you receive, you have already become an insurance company employee. Send your bills to Medicare and Medicaid, and you're on the government payroll. But bill your patient for professional fees, shifting the burden of responsibility to the man who receives treatment, and another link in the doctor-patient relation has been forged.

HEALTH INSURANCE

The age of health insurance is upon us, salvation of the surgeon, hope of the hospital, and penance of the doctor's overworked aide. Rare is the patient who pays his own way. Each coughing infant, wheezing oldster, and aching arthritic has a form attached. Study these documents carefully. The questions are loaded, and oversights can explode into financial crisis for the patient and embarrassment for the physician.

"What was the date of onset of the illness?" Let's start with a tricky one. Miss Insurance Clerk isn't expressing idle curiosity. Note that she wants the date of Mr. Patient's first symptoms, not the day he finally arrived in your office. Why? There's only one good reason for this question on the form: If symptoms antedate the effective date of policy coverage, the insurance company disclaims responsibility. Date that recently changing nevus you removed back to the patient's childhood and the insurance company may reply, "Oh, no. It's not our problem." Keep your answers pertinent, describe recent developments, and ignore irrelevant past history.

"Does the patient have other health insurance?" Here's another loaded question. Filling in two forms? Tempted to check both affirmative? Then brace for a squabble, as each financial giant claims responsibility only after the other has tendered his maximum payment.

"What is the diagnosis?" Usually there's little trouble here—as long as you describe an ailment. Tom Smith may have suffered with dandruff and flatfeet, prompting a comprehensive physical examination. If you answer "routine physical examination" Tom's insurance benefits may evaporate. On the other hand, if you tell Miss Insurance Clerk about Tom's seborrhea of the scalp and pes planus, your patient may realize a small return on his whopping annual premium.

"What were the dates of partial and total disability?" Sometimes health insurance claims involve disability riders. It's really hard to conjure up disability dates for preschool infants and housewives, even when the form inquires. For working men, it's easier—related to his return to light and full duties. Are you in doubt about exact dates? Don't estimate. Telephone the patient. If you're pretty sure the question is not applicable—little Mary Smith's tonsillitis is unlikely to yield disability payments—leave that section blank. If Miss Insurance Clerk is really interested, she'll send a note.

"What is your fee for professional services?" Here's where attention to clerical detail pays off. Itemize your charges, breaking down lump sums into details, including office visit, throat culture, blood test, and x-ray. Lump-sum billing is expediently reduced to the company's single-office-call allowance, but itemized charges are hard to fault.

"Doctor, I sure hope you get your money from the insurance company." Here's a dangerous attitude, and a few words of explanation are in order. "Mr. Patient, fees for professional services will be billed to your account. Any insurance payments received will be credited, but in the end, we look to you for payment." Certainly, your office will labor over forms, assisting the patient in every way to obtain insurance payments. But when claims have been rejected and protests ignored, it's up to Mr. Patient to dig deep in his pocket.

Don't pull out the rug from under your aide with such statements as, "Don't worry. Insurance will cover everything." In effect, you've made a contract. A thoughtless word guaranteeing insurance coverage can cause embarrassment if the claim is rejected and may negate your patient's personal responsibility for your fee.

Must you accept insurance company payments as your total fee? Of course not. At this writing, the doctor is still a free agent, free to determine his own fair and reasonable fees. Complete the insurance form, detail your charges for professional care, credit receipts to your patient's account, and bill him for the difference.

MEDICAID AND WELFARE

Up and down bounce eligibility requirements. Families leap on and off the Medicaid bandwagon, clutching multicolored cards. Exceptions abound. Some cards allow hospital care only. Others disclaim responsibility for preventive care. And many, if examined closely, expired yesterday. What's the doctor to do?

Need you accept Medicaid-welfare payments? Many doctors don't. Are they greedy, abandoning indigent patients to the ravages of disease? I don't think so. Since the time of Hippocrates, physicians have treated the indigent as well as the affluent, charging what the patient could comfortably afford. Many times payment was a word of thanks and a promise for the future. Then came welfare; the government benevolently assumed responsibility for medical care of the "medically indigent." Oh happy day. The doctor will finally be paid. But soon the honeymoon was over. A welter of forms, bureaucratic red tape, autocratic directives, and an unhealthy aversion to check-writing caused a rift between the government and physicians. Disillusioned, many doctors returned to the traditional "pay me when and if you can" medical care of the indigent.

Let's return to the practical question: Need you accept Medicaid-welfare payments? Surgeons are stuck; so are most physicians who charge large fees for single procedures. The patient who qualifies for welfare payments usually can't afford a $350 cholecystectomy. But in the office, it's a different story. Many office based physicians continue to care for Medicaid-welfare patients, charging reduced (or usual) fees. A $5 or $8 office visit every few months won't bankrupt the welfare family. Write Medicaid prescriptions when your sample drawer runs low. At year's end, your accountant may point out the folly of your ways and insist that welfare payments would increase your gross income, but in my opinion, the dignity of my patients' paying their own way is worth more than a few dollars.

What fee should you charge the Medicaid-welfare Department? If you decide to accept payments, bill the agency your full fee. Of course, you know *their* fee schedule is probably about half yours. And that reduced fee, barely covering overhead, is all they're going to pay. Bill your full fee, anyhow. Somewhere, out there, in the vast network of communicating computers your fee profile is in a state of evolution. Bill the Welfare Department reduced fees, and those bargain rates are fed into the computer and averaged against your true charges, producing a distorted, artifically low fee profile.

Welfare-Medicaid prescriptions are a pain in the hand; writer's cramp results from repetitive prescription copying, necessitated by bureaucratic fiat. Soon, Mr. Welfare learns that aspirin, Ace bandages, Band-Aids, and Milk of Magnesia are free, "when prescribed" by the doctor. In he comes with his shopping list, with no illness other than avarice. Speed this patient's office visit by teaching your nurse to transcribe prescriptions, using the prescription-renewal form illustrated in Chapter 21. Insist that Mr. Welfare come to the office in person to pick up his prescriptions. And wrestle with your conscience concerning the propriety of stocking his home medicine cabinet with prescription Band-Aids.

When writing welfare-Medicaid prescriptions, and indeed, all prescriptions, specify the number of refills, be it once, 20 times, or no refill. But don't use the designation "p.r.n." indicating renewal as needed. Indefinite and confusing, the p.r.n. refillable prescription means one refill to the first pharmacist, indefinite refills to the next, and no refill to the third.

MEDICARE

Despite initial opposition by organized medicine, Medicare has become part of the American way of life. Taken as a whole, the program has succeeded—preventing catastrophic illness from bankrupting senior citizens.

Form SSA-1490 is the key to Medicare payments. Form SSA-1490, more than any other form, must be completed accurately; few elderly patients can conquer their half of the form without mishap, and your aide will save many hours of work if she checks your elderly patient's data before he leaves the office.

Part 1 of Form SSA-1490 is the patient's half—containing his name, health insurance claim number, mailing address, description of his illness, information concerning other health insurance or state medical assistance, signature, and date.

Double-check the health insurance claim numbers (item 2); a mix-up here can delay processing of the claim. The patient's description of his illness (item 4) must be completed if the doctor does not fill in part II of the form. If the senior citizen has other medical insurance or receives Medicaid benefits, enter the agency and identification number in item 5.

Part II is the physician's half of the form. In theory, part II need not be completed if detailed statements are attached, including all information necessary to process the Medicare claim. (As described in Chapter 17, your office charge slip should include all data necessary.) In practice, the completion of part II, at least in skeleton form, speeds payment considerably. Medicare clerks are accustomed to processing data in the SSA-1490 format. Let them wrestle with your usual office statement and confusion may occur. You may add your office bill for completeness, but complete item 7A showing dates of service, item 7B showing place of service, item 7C describing procedures and services, item 7D relating the nature of illness or injury, and most important, item 7E showing charges. Under no circum tances should you omit item 9, the total charges. Here's where the clerk looks first. Then, if your information is easily translated into computerese, the all-knowing electronic wizard may reward you with a payment check.

Should you accept Medicare payments? One key to this riddle is found on the back of Form SSA-1490: "Under this method (assignment), the doctor agrees to accept the charge determination of the Medicare carrier as the full charge." The Medicare fee schedule is always a few years behind the times, the inevitable result of computing fees retrospectively, lumping recently submitted data with old facts in a memory bank. Accept assignment, and the way is paved for easy payment—at bargain rates. If you provide a high-priced service that yields an income to match, assignment of Medicare benefits may be the right road for you.

How about the office-based physician, his family fed on income derived from tonsillitis, flu, and aching backs, supplemented by a few hospital patients and fewer house calls? Here the road to Medicare payments is full of potholes. Medicare billing for the single office or house call is time-consuming, both for your aide and the Medicare clerk; the latter often expresses her displeasure with annoying petty requests for additional information. By the time your final (and administratively reduced) fee is paid, the value of clerical services expended exceeds the amount of the check. Small wonder that most office-based physicians insist upon the individual patient's responsibility for his medical bills and cheerfully assist oldsters in the completion of SSA-1490.

Can you have your cake and eat it too? Yes, you can. You can bill old Mrs. Johnson this month and accept assignment the next. Many doctors decline assignment in the office, but accept direct Medicare payment for large hospital bills truly beyond the means of elderly patients.

Your fee profile, is it myth or reality? Yes, Virginia, there really is a fee profile. Somewhere, out there on a reel of tape in some distant memory bank, is your fee profile. Probably you'll never see it, a crowning paradox of bureaucracy. "But," says Medicare, "if doctors were allowed to see their profiles, they would compare them and set fees."

As the specter of federal fee controls casts a pall over the profession, the individual doctor's fee profile becomes his sanctuary. Guard your fee profile; protect it carefully. When you consider doing a senior citizen a favor by charging a reduced fee, remember that that bargain fee is averaged into your fee profile. Someday soon, you may be stuck with it. Medicare has taken the joy out of small favors; they may return to haunt you in years to come.

WORKMEN'S COMPENSATION

Workmen's Compensation legislation has removed the burden of proof from employees, negated the need for establishing liability, and assured that on-the-job injuries receive competent medical care at no cost to the worker. Funded by private insurance companies, embraced by the medical profession, this is social legislation at its most creative.

Of course, whenever insurance companies and agencies enter the picture, forms are devised to bring order to data. Understand your state's Workmen's Compensation form and guide its completion to assure proper benefits to the injured employee and prompt payment to the doctor.

"Describe the injury completely," relating its occurrence to employment. Specify the date, time, and circumstances surrounding the accident. Negligence is not a factor; the sole criterion for Workmen's Compensation acceptance is an on-the-job injury.

"Is there a history of previous injury?" Here's danger. The patient with a history of recurrent low back ache may have trouble relating his present acute sacroiliac strain to his present employment. Of course, you must include details of possible previous injuries, and in these cases, take special pains to document the authenticity of today's injury.

"What treatment was provided?" Include everything, including sutures, tetanus booster, physical therapy, and, most important, your specific recommendation concerning work. The professional statement of fees submitted with the Workmen's Compensation form must correlate with the treatment described.

"May the injury result in permanent loss of function or disfigurement, yes or no?" This is often a difficult question, particularly in the early weeks of treatment. Yes or no answers are fine for computers, but the best reply may be "maybe." If so, write it in, until the final result of treatment is known.

"Has the patient been referred for vocational rehabilitation?" Occasionally, this question can trip you up. Certainly irrelevant in short-term lacerations and sprains, the question of vocational rehabilitation achieves significance in long-term disability—the carpenter with an injured hand or the salesclerk with painful ambulation. An unsympathetic referee, evaluating a chronically disabled employee, may frown on your failure to obtain vocational rehabilitation counseling and use this excuse to reduce payments. I know; it happened to one of my patients.

"When can the patient return to work?" This is the *raison d'être* of treatment under the Workmen's Compensation Act. Once accepted, the case must be pursued at least until the patient returns to work. As the sprained ankle heals, the swelling subsides, and the cane is discarded, it's time to ask, "Do you feel ready to go back to work?" Discuss with your patient his specific duties, considering his injuries in relation to his activities. When you agree, pick a day, and write it in your records, underlined for speedy location by your secretary when she completes the form. In many cases, it is therapeutic for the patient to watch you write the date. It seals the bargain; and caution him to call if he's unable to resume employment on the date agreed.

Sometimes it takes a little pressure to get that lingering compensation case back to work. "Doctor, I don't think I'm ready to go back to work yet. My back still hurts at times." But you think he's ready. How about part-time work, light work, just a few hours a day—anything to get him back on the job. Still resists? Then discuss with your reluctant workman the consequences of unduly prolonged compensation cases. "Now, Tom, if we wind up the case, get you back to work, and submit a final report, there should be no difficulty with the claim. But if the case drags on, the insurance company may question the claim, possibly involving a hearing with lawyers, adjusters, and so forth. Don't you think we could get you back to work soon? How about Monday?"

When your slow-to-respond compensation patient returns to work, hold your breath, and hold your "final" report a few weeks, lest he suffer a relapse. Once you have submitted a final report, the insurance company closes its books on the case. And reopening a "closed" compensation case is about as easy as making water flow uphill.

While on the subject of reopening old compensation cases, here's another tip: Do you have a patient with a job-related acute low back strain? "Doctor, I'm sure this all began with the injury 3 years ago. I thought I was well. The case was closed, and then the pain came back." Stifle the urge to pursue the old case. Reams of forms are only the first step; lawyers and hearings—all unnecessary—often follow. Simply open a new case. Complete the form, describing the recent injury and being careful to include the past history of similar complaints. Explain why the new injury is a distinct entity, the direct result of his current employment. It is 10 times easier to open a new compensation case than to reopen a closed one.

Is there a lawyer on the case? Workmen's Compensation cases may be clouded by negligence, permanent disability, and other grounds for litigation. Are you the personal physician for such a claimant? Then help your patient and his attorney: Send the attorney a photocopy of each report sent to the insurance carrier. Give your patient's lawyer a fighting chance. Compensation insurance carriers receive thousands of reports daily. Your critical report, carefully composed, detailing your patient's treatment was mailed 3 weeks ago. Now you have been notified of a hearing a few days hence. Don't be surprised if the insurance company "can't find" or "never received" your crucial report. But at the hearing, you're ready: Your patient's lawyer has a copy. So do you. The "lost" report can be admitted as evidence.

Bills to compensation insurance carriers are usually paid promptly, but some bills, like some reports, get lost. Or perhaps they are handled by inaction. Send monthly statements to your Workmen's Compensation carriers, just as you do your other patients. Of course, enclose an up-to-date progress report. Is the account overdue? Are your statements being filed and forgotten? Then send a query to the insurance carrier with a copy to your state Workmen's Compensation Board.

Still no payment? Is the insurance company ignoring your existence? Then bypass the insurance carrier and send a note of protest to the Director of your state's Workmen's Compensation Board. Results should follow swiftly.

LIFE INSURANCE COMPANIES

The giant life insurance companies are more stable than the United States Government. They show a profit annually. Only strict actuarial analysis of applicant risk can sustain this record, and in the end, the data submitted concerning an applicant come from the office of a practicing physician.

Set your own fee for insurance medical examinations. Doctors who offer good reports are scarce. The submitted application is a legal document, and a small percentage of original applications will eventually end in litigation. The prompt completion of a legible, accurate, legally defensible report is well worth your fee. Nine out of ten companies will pay it happily. The mechanism? Cross out the $15 preprinted fee on the voucher and substitute your own. How about those forms with a pre-stamped check, designed to be detached and cashed? Fine. Bank the check and bill the insurance company for the balance. My office sends statements to various insurance companies monthly; usually they are paid promptly if the claim is adequately documented, including date, name of applicant, service performed, and very important for the bookkeeping department, the company's applicant identification number.

Don't allow insurance salesmen to make appointments for medical examinations. This should be a strict rule. Appointments are made only by the patient (applicant). Commission-hungry salesmen use medical appointments as a pressure gimmick to force a sale. When the prospective insurance buyer gets cold feet, he ignores both the salesman's pleas and the medical examination appointment made by the salesman. And there you are, with an empty half-hour on your hands and egg on your face.

The applicant arriving for an insurance medical examination should bring the necessary forms and urine container. This should be another rigid dictum. Make exceptions and you'll be sorry. Here's why: During the course of a year, you may perform insurance medical examinations for as many as 15 or 20 companies, each with its own forms, mailing envelopes, and urine specimen containers. Act as a repository for these supplies for that many companies, and you'll need an extra storeroom to handle the volume. Also, store these supplies, and you have assumed responsibility for keeping up the stock. Then, when Mr. Applicant arrives for his medical examination for the Lastgasp Insurance Company and you are fresh out of Lastgasp urine specimen bottles, you look pretty foolish. Shift responsibility to the applicant and the salesman by insisting that they bring in all paraphernalia for the examination.

As mentioned above, the insurance medical examination form is a legal document, permanently filed with the original application and subject to review if discrepancies become apparent. As with any legal document, extra care is needed. Print clearly, using a black pen (these records will be photostated); erasures are prohibited. If an error is made, correct by drawing a single line through the incorrect entry, adding your initials and date. Be sure to obtain the patient's signature, usually in two places, the first certifying the accuracy of the medical history and the second authorizing the release of any and all medical records to the company.

A photostatic copy of the record release may arrive in your office a few weeks later, stapled to a request for medical information. The busy medical office fields a few such requests every week. Most follow a standard format, requesting details of each patient visit in your applicant's record—date of visit, symptoms, pertinent physical findings, duration of the illness, diagnosis, treatment, and pertinent laboratory tests. A narrative report is acceptable and some companies offer a toll-free telephone number for dictation. Insurance companies rely upon accurate informative reports and are willing to pay for them. The usual fee is $10, but most companies will go higher for extensive reports, supplemented by photocopies of data from your records.

Some companies send their standard form with a preprinted $3 or $5 check. Complete the form, bank the check, and bill the insurance company for the balance by posting the amount due on a ledger card, mailed each month with your usual bills.

An occasional cut-rate insurance company submits requests for medical information with no intention of paying for your time. The covering letter usually mentions your patient's fervent desire for the insurance and the wish that you will perform this service as a favor. Most insurance companies are considerably more affluent than the practicing physician; charity is for paupers. For $10, your local printer will run off

1000 index cards describing your policy concerning requests for medical information (Fig. 22–1). Staple your card to the form, stuff it back into the generously provided stamped envelope, and return it to the company. Watch the request come home again, this time with a $10 check.

Robert B. Taylor, M.D.
66 Forest Glen Road
New Paltz, New York 12561

Gentlemen:

    My office charges a clerical fee of ten dollars to cover services involved in preparing reports of this type.

    You may re-submit your form along with a check for ten dollars.

Yours very truly,
Dr. Taylor

Fig. 22–1. Preprinted form stating fee policy in regard to insurance reports.

Not all news is good news. Sometimes you must submit an adverse medical report. A description of your patient's long-forgotten episode of paroxysmal atrial tachycardia or childhood glomerulonephritis may dash his chances of purchasing reasonably priced life insurance—forever. Price fixing is prohibited, but insurance companies are allowed to exchange information freely, and they do. A single unfavorable medical report goes into the computer and is spewed forth whenever the patient applies for insurance again. Play fair with him. Inform your patient of the report you must prepare and the possible consequences. Let him see the report, if appropriate. Then submit it only with his approval.

DISABILITY INSURANCE

Here's where Mr. Patient is paid for not being well, sometimes by a governmental agency and other times by his private insurance carrier. Dates of partial and total disability are of paramount importance here.

Don't accept the disability claim form until Mr. Patient has filled in "his part," including the dates he last worked and first returned to work. Compare these dates with your entries to avoid embarrassing discrepancies.

"Was the injury or illness related to employment?" Watch this one.

An affirmative answer, no matter how tenuous the relation, will probably result in a Workmen's Compensation claim.

"If still disabled, when do you expect the patient to return to work?" Be generous here. Estimate a 2-week disability, and a 3-month convalescence will raise eyebrows at the company home office. On the other hand, a 6-week estimate of disability, followed by a return to work at the end of 1 month, will certainly be favorably received.

Tell your aide to put disability forms at the top of the pile. These documents mean money in the patient's pocket, vitally important to disabled patients whose other income may be lacking. In fact, some disability forms have short time limits and are rendered invalid if received late. So, get your disability forms out fast; Mr. Patient's family needs grocery money.

Those pesky third parties are a fact of modern medical practice, existing in symbiosis with physicians. We provide the medical care; they have the money. Deal with them honestly, frankly, and from a position of strength—and claims will be paid fully. Don't let insurance companies intimidate you. Until they learn to practice medicine, they need you more than you need them.

References and Suggestions for Further Reading

1. Allied Health Personnel: Ad Hoc Committee on Allied Health Personnel. Washington, D C, National Academy of Sciences, 1969.

2. Bogdonoff M D: Concern about patient care. Arch Intern Med 123:719–721, 1969.

3. Falk I S: Beyond Medicare. J Public Health 59:608–623, 1969.

4. Fuchs V R: The growing demand for medical care. N Engl J Med 279:190–195, 1968.

5. Gooche G W, Taylor R B: We refuse Medicaid money. Physician's Management 12:3 p. 44–47 March 1972.

6. Levey S: A perspective on Medicaid. N Engl J Med 281:297–301, 1969.

7. McBride E D: Disability Evaluation and Principles of Treatment of Compensable Injuries. Philadelphia, Lippincott, 1963.

8. Shannon J A: Medicine, public policy and the private sector. N Engl J Med 281:135–141, 1969.

9. Sheppard J D: The doctor's "business condition." Postgrad Med 47:202–207, 1970.

10. Task Force on Prescription Drugs. Washington, D C, U S Dept Health, Education, Welfare, 1969.

11. Taylor R B: Games Medicare people play. Physician's Management 11:56–57, 1971.

12. White K L: Personal incentives, professional standards and public accountability for health care. Hospitals 42:74–78, 1968.

23

Through the Medicolegal Jungle

He that goes to law holds a wolf by the ears.

Robert Burton
(1577–1640)

As the doctor lightheartedly makes his daily rounds, hidden eyes are watching. The wolf, often disguised in sheep's clothing, surveys every move. One misstep—a slip of the knife, a bungled telephone call, an angry word to a patient—can fell the doctor, leaving him helpless, the wolf at his throat. Carefully chart your course through the medicolegal jungle. Guard your flanks with good doctor-patient relations, your back with exemplary records, and be wary of the malpractice traps in your own office.

CHART A CLEAR PATH THROUGH THE MEDICOLEGAL JUNGLE

A first-rate doctor-patient relationship is the best professional liability insurance. The patient who appreciates that his doctor "did his best" will rarely sue. A puzzling problem? A poor result? A permanent disability? All are acceptable when patient and doctor agree that everyone put forth their top efforts, exercising their best judgment at the time.

We could take a lesson from cultists and quacks. They *take care* of their patients. Perhaps they act from fright, but the message of sincere concern comes through. When things go wrong, the quack is quick to respond, offering solace if not good medical care.

Contrast the quack with John Q. Specialist, M.D., presently mired in his third professional liability suit in 5 years. Dr. Specialist's training can't be faulted, his clinical judgment is (usually) flawless. But things go wrong. They always do. And when trouble strikes, Dr. Specialist arrogantly proclaims the superiority of his treatment, implies that the complication is a demonstration of patient ingratitude, brushes off inquiries from worried family members, and hides behind his answering service. Dr. John Q. Specialist may offer the best medical care in the state, but his professional liability insurance rates are 10 times than those of the quacks—testimony to the superior prophylactic capabilities of the good doctor-patient relationship.

Trouble may begin when you try to do too much. Do you squeeze in, double, work through lunch, and stay late? Or worse, do you skip electrocardiography, x-rays, blood tests, or pelvic examinations because the press of patients limits time? The days when cases turn sour are usually days when you have seen more patients than your office is geared to handle. Rushed, you occasionally neglect details, and the seed of professional liability is sown.

Refrain from procedures beyond your competence. Don't start anything you can't finish. The practicing physician, the supreme individualist, lives the fantasy of total competence in all areas of medicine and surgery. Isn't that what his medical license says? But in practice, the physician who encounters one or two Colles' fractures yearly should refer those few to an orthopedic surgeon. Sure, he reduced a few in medical school. But unless he performs a procedure regularly, the doctor loses familiarity. His radar doesn't register the early warning of complications. Problems result and litigation may follow. Do what you do best; refer the rest.

Office pitfalls are everywhere. Tomorrow, when you have a spare moment, look around. Are your medication samples outdated? Are your autoclaved instruments really sterile? Are your hot packs too hot? Is there a rickety chair in your waiting room? Ice in the parking lot? And don't forget climbing infants who can find hazards in areas safe for adults.

How about the attitude of your aides? Are they arrogant? Overbearing? A trifle careless? Or do they communicate a genuine interest in the patients' welfare? Examine your own attitudes—your aides will reflect your concern for or disdain of patients. A harsh word, a subtle rebuff, can undo hours of counseling and leave the patient convinced that "the doctor's office really doesn't care."

MEDICOLEGAL TRAPS

Telephone advice can return to haunt you. Some say the doctor should never offer advice over the telephone. Unrealistic, say I. Infant-feeding problems, a patient's progress report, and minor common colds are amenable to telephone therapy. But you must know your patient. Some mothers consult the doctor only when the child is *in extremis;* a call from such a woman should be followed by examination of the youngster. Other mothers call about every sniffle, and constructive telephone advice can increase self-reliance.

Sometimes the key is finding out what the patient has in mind. What does he really want—a telephoned prescription for a decongestant, an office visit, or referral to a specialist? Beside providing good medical care, the goal of therapy is to satisfy the patient—difficult to do without learning the patient's desire.

Telephone calls from unknown patients are particularly hazardous. Without knowledge of the patient's judgment, evaluation is difficult. Most telephone calls from new patients should prompt an office visit, firmly establishing the doctor-patient relation and allowing you to size up your new charge.

Offer no telephone advice unless you plan to accept responsibility for the new patient. Does the patient reside many miles away? Are your appointments booked for 2 weeks hence? Perhaps your practice is closed. Then politely inform the unknown caller that you cannot accept his case. Don't solicit historical data. Don't offer a telephone diagnosis. And most important, don't suggest interim or definitive therapy. Stand your ground firmly, explain that you cannot accept the case, and suggest that he call another physician or go directly to the hospital emergency room.

Telephone advice should be recorded. In the office, a call should not be accepted or returned until your aide has placed the patient's folder in front of you. The telephone call entry should include the date, the notation that advice was rendered over the telephone and not in the office, the patient's complaints, and your recommendations, including specific advice concerning follow-up "if things don't go as expected." Color-code your notes: I record office-visit notations in black ink and telephone conversations in blue. How about that telephone conversation from your home? Make a note or record on tape and transfer it to the patient's clinical record in the morning. Some physicians use note pads; the conversation is recorded at the desk or at home and the tear-off slip taped to the telephone page in the clinical record.

The 3 A.M. telephone call is a medicolegal trap. Groggy, floundering in the dark to silence an insistently ringing phone, the physician tries to rub sleep from his eyes. On the line is a patient or nurse, wide awake and coherent. Suddenly, the sleepy doctor is called upon for a life-or-death decision. Ludicrous errors have resulted—heat applied to cold ischemic feet or orders for intramuscular milk of magnesia—usually, but not always, questioned by the wide-awake party. When that early morning telephone call beckons, wake up. Turn on the light. Sit up. Transfer the call to another room. Check a textbook. Whatever you do, keep talking, asking questions, and defer definitive recommendations until you wake up! Then compose a written note, detailing the conversation and add it to the patient's record in the morning.

Missed appointments should be noted. The patient with bronchitis who failed to keep his follow-up appointment, the ulcer victim who spurned his recheck visit, and the life insurance applicant who never found his way to your office should all have notations in their clinical records. Note also when George Smith calls to report that his back strain has recovered and he wants to cancel his appointment tomorrow. Some day, years from now, his failure to keep his scheduled appointment may become important to an insurance company, a lawyer, or you.

Is a written consent necessary for office surgery? Many say it is and dutifully demand signatures before repairing minor lacerations or removing an ugly mole. Certainly, the hospital demands written acquiescence for any procedure more profound than a penicillin injection, and in years to come, simple immunizations may have to be preceded by ritual consent signing. How about procedures in the office? Lawyers may disagree, but in a family practice, I consider the patient's submission to the procedure to be implied consent. Without the patient's approval, no nevus is removable and no laceration reparable. No, I don't use consent forms for office surgery, and while results aren't always as good as I might hope, no patient has ever complained that the procedure was performed without his approval.

X-rays are tangible documentation of your observations. Fluoroscopic images can't be brought to court. When evaluating a traumatic injury, particularly when liability is involved, take x-rays, don't fluoroscope. And when the case involves potential liability, as an auto accident or a fall in a department store, x-ray every painful area. When the plaintiff's case comes to trial, you will bless your foresight.

Medical treatment of a famous person may subject the doctor to the inquisition of the press. The popular athlete, renowned statesman, or cinema sex symbol falls prey to disease of the flesh. And the illness is news. So is the doctor. Here are some tips to guide your dealings with reporters:

1. Check your county medical society's press-release guide. What do your colleagues consider a prudent report to the fourth estate?
2. Is your patient truly in the public domain? If so, he is considered fair prey for reporters, and a candid press release may preserve your privacy and eliminate multiple annoying home telephone calls.
3. Carefully compose your press release and review it with the patient or his representative. Be sure you all agree on form and content before it is submitted to the waiting reporters. Get that approval in writing.
4. Release "just the facts." That means first-hand knowledge, not hearsay, gossip, or speculation. Exactly when did the accident occur? What were the exact injuries? How long was the patient in the operating room? Parry leading questions with a stone-faced "no comment."
5. State the patient's condition in general terms—good, fair, poor, or critical. Be guarded in your prognosis, and shun imaginative predictions.

WILL YOUR RECORDS HOLD UP IN COURT?

Legible, well-organized records enhance the doctor's courtroom image. Dog-eared cards with coffee stains convey a courtroom impression of sloppiness, an impression lawyers and jurors assign to the card-bearer himself. Many an outstanding physician has appeared foolish on the witness stand, searching for a simple fact in his pile of cards. He shuffles, fumbles, and drops them on the floor. Jurors try hard not to snicker, and the value of his testimony lies strewn on the floor with the smudged cards.

Hearsay evidence can creep into your records. Entries made by nurses and aides, accurate though they may be, might be questioned by a hostile attorney. "Doctor, did *you* perform the visual acuity test?" Of course, you didn't; your office nurse tested the vision and recorded the result in the patient's clinical record—all quite proper. But she isn't there in court. If the patient's visual acuity is critical to an automobile liability case, a sharp lawyer may contest the admissibility of the evidence. The doctor didn't test the patient himself, and more to the point, the notation is in someone else's handwriting. How to solve the problem? Must the doctor make all chart entries? No, as long as the doctor is careful to initial and date all employee record entries on liability cases, another check-point in preparation for court testimony.

Erasures can invalidate your records. Certainly, we all make clerical errors. The wrong accident date is recorded, the wrong chart is pulled, or a last minute medication change is made. Should you scratch out the error or obliterate with opaquing fluid? No. There's only one legal way to correct chart errors. A single straight line is drawn through the incorrect entry and initialed and dated by the person making the correction.

Your office record may be shown or read to the court as you shrink into the witness chair. Often highly personal and colorful, office records are a privileged communication between patient and doctor—until litigation results. Then the court can subpoena your record, leaving your office to struggle with photocopies, while the original thumb-marked folder rests ceremoniously in court. Prepare records that will do you credit when your day in court arrives.

Physicians sometimes unwittingly submit their records as evidence. Obligingly, Dr. Brown dictated detailed reports to the insurance company and lawyers. Now he's on the witness stand, testifying to supplement his neat typewritten reports. The attorney asks a question. Dr. Brown brings out his office record, "to refresh his memory." Bang! The record has become evidence. Either attorney may request to view the record, including asking for a recess to examine its contents thoroughly. If the office folder has weak spots, a hostile attorney, trained to dissect medical records, will spot them faster than any physician. Dr. Brown may be in for trouble—trouble of his own making.

LAWYERS NEED RECORDS, TOO

Most litigation cases involve automobile mishaps or other accidental injuries. To act effectively, your patient's lawyer needs accurate information. The clinical notation concerning every injury examined in the office should have the following details:

1. The date, time, and place of the injury.
2. If an automobile accident, how many vehicles were involved?
3. Where was the patient at the time of the accident? Right front seat passenger, driver of the automobile, or walking along the sidewalk?

4. How did the accident happen? Use the patient's exact words here, identifying his statements in quotes.
5. What complaints does the patient have? Where does he hurt? List every complaint however trivial it might appear.

Personal injury cases involving liability often drag on for years. Imagine your consternation upon receiving a request for a detailed report concerning a patient who visited once for an apparently trivial injury and never returned. Avoid such situations by following all liability cases until the patient is well and the litigation terminated. Do you think the injuries are minor? Prompt recovery expected? Nevertheless, insist that the victim return for reexamination. That second visit of the accident victim is often more revealing than the first—increased pain, new complaints, and a lawyer's business card. Follow your accident cases to completion, and you'll be blessed with adequate records when the case comes to court.

Disfiguring injuries change with time. The emotional scars of a deep jagged laceration may persist years after the skin is healed. When the case is brought before a jury several years from now, your patient's lawyer would trade his briefcase for an accurate drawing or, even better, a photograph of the injuries. A brief sketch in your clinical record is a help. If you're a camera buff, use your expensive toy to provide your patient with a permanent record of his injuries.

Reports to lawyers must be complete. Many will be introduced in court as evidence. The proper legal report includes a visit-by-visit record of the patient's complaints, your physical findings, and recommended therapy. Here's a check list to evaluate your medical reports to attorneys:

1. Date, time, and place of accident
2. Patient's description of accident
3. Date patient first reported to you for treatment
4. Visit-by-visit synopsis of his progress
5. Your diagnoses—complete, specific, and anatomic
6. The recommended therapy, including medication, physical therapy, and activity permitted
7. The patient's disability, both partial and total
8. Your prognosis, as detailed as reasonable, allowing room for possible setbacks
9. The statement of professional fees, detailed and itemized
10. The physician's signature

Charge the attorney for your medical report. A well-composed report takes at least an hour to complete. The minimal charge for a legal document is $25. Higher fees are in order when extra time is spent. The fee paid for a medical report is part of the attorney's cost of doing business and is usually cheerfully forwarded in return for a professional-quality report. An occasional attorney instructs your patient, "Tell your doctor to send me a report." Don't do it, for two reasons. First, it's unprofessional, and lacks the protocol of a formal request for records. In fact, the attorney may only have requested a statement of disability or professional fees. You don't really know what he wants. Second, the specific request for a medical report, received from an attorney, implies that the lawyer will pay for your efforts. Feel guilty about charging for reports? Consider what attorneys charge *you* for completing a few forms.

Some attorneys refuse to pay for medical reports—most commonly these are out-of-town barristers with whom you are unlikely ever to do business again. With known tightwads or unknown out-of-town attorneys, you have two choices. With the patient's approval, the cost of the medical report may be added to his bill, possibly to be paid by the insurance company in the end. Do you feel strongly that the lawyer should pay his own way? Then insist upon advance payment: "Dear Sir: The medical report you requested concerning Mr. John Patient will be forthcoming upon receipt of your check for $25 in payment for my time in preparation of this document. Thank you."

YOUR DAY IN COURT

Rest assured, your day will come. Few physicians in active practice can escape an occasional court appearance. Although he occasionally appears as an expert witness, the practicing physician is usually summoned to give testimony relative to his treatment of an injured victim.

When informed by a lawyer that your patient's case is coming to court and your testimony will be needed, here are a few tips. Ask if your testimony can be taken as a deposition. Admissible as evidence, the deposition can be taken at your convenience—eliminating a lost day in the office. Without the emotionally charged drama of the courtroom, many physicians can provide more lucid testimony by deposition than on the witness stand.

"No, Doctor, this case will call for your testimony on the witness stand." If so, the lawyer will (or should) insist upon a consultation before the case begins. He will preview some questions he plans to ask in court, hoping to unearth the explosive answer in his office rather than the courtroom. At the conference, he will explain the hypothetical question: Assuming certain facts concerning the accident, in your professional opinion, could the patient's present pain and suffering reasonably be attributed to the injury? Of course, he will go into much more detail, often rambling for several paragraphs. Listen carefully in his office; you may miss some of it in court. A properly prepared hypothetical question is answered with a single word, "Yes."

While conferring with the attorney, extract two promises. First, insist that your testimony be delivered at a specified hour, eliminating a long wait in the court anteroom. Second, request that your arrival be properly timed. Many an eager attorney has scheduled the doctor's arrival at a moment calculated to disrupt the testimony of the opposition's key witness or to force an earlier hearing of the case, hoping the judge will accede to the physician's press of time. Such scheduling is no accident, but the conniving of clever attorneys, using physicians as pawns.

Your court testimony warrants a fee. Charge for your time. If your testimony involves a half day lost from the office, your fee should be a half day's gross income. If the court appearance results in the loss of a full day's income in the office, that's your fee.

During testimony, an attorney may wheel, point a finger at you, and inquire, "Doctor, are you being paid for your testimony?" The correct answer? "No, but I will submit a statement for my time in court today."

Prepare for your court appearance as you would for a medical examination. Your testimony on the witness stand is indeed a test; the court is evaluating your medical knowledge, appearance, and demeanor.

Study your records. Review everything, including the office progress notes, laboratory reports, x-rays, and hospital records. Is the case long and involved? Perhaps a brief outline will bring it into focus. Does the case hinge on a single medical fact? Then study. You will be quizzed. Make sure your information is up-to-date.

How about medical textbooks? Should you quote them? I wouldn't. Your erudition may amaze the jury, but lawyers know all the tricks. Claim familiarity with a medical text, and a hostile attorney may make a dunce of you. Stick to your own facts and opinions. Leave quotations to authors.

Overstated qualifications can boomerang. Be modest. If you're a general practitioner, say so, without implying expertise in specialized areas. A humble statement of qualifications paves the way for ducking tricky questions. "I'm sorry, I'm a family physician. You'd better ask a specialist that question."

Remain impartial. Don't take sides. In your heart, you may believe your patient has a valid case and deserves a generous award. But leave your emotions at home. Stick to facts and present them untainted with bias.

Don't be rattled by loaded questions. "Doctor, have you and the plaintiff's lawyer discussed your testimony?" Correct answer? "Yes, we had a conference yesterday, and the case was discussed in detail." No judge would expect you to testify without a discussion with the patient's attorney, and a negative answer will only set the stage for a barrage of embarrassing questions, extracting the contradictory testimony that you have, indeed, conferred with your patient's lawyer.

"Never volunteer" they say in the army. The same holds true for court testimony. Both attorneys have evolved a line of questioning to bring out the salient facts. Answer their questions directly, and the true story will eventually emerge.

Don't be trapped into "yes or no" answers when a qualification is needed. Many queries are carefully couched to evoke a slanted answer if the doctor is restricted to a yes or no reply. Ignore this and respond briefly, but in your own words.

Speak up. Don't mumble. Address your answers to the jury, not the judge or the plaintiff. Notice courtroom lawyers. They stand well away from the witness, calling for forceful audible replies.

Dress conservatively. Don't dazzle the jury with your sartorial splendor. During a medical convention, a hotel employee was once heard to remark, "You can always tell the doctors. Their coats and trousers don't match." Appear in court wearing a dignified business suit and a quiet tie. You are a respected member of an honored profession. Look the part.

HOW DOES A PROFESSIONAL LIABILITY SUIT BEGIN?

Things go wrong, and the seed of discontent is sown. But unless nurtured by arrogance, hostility, and indifference, it will wither and die. But, if sown in fertile ground, nourished by words of criticism, and warmed by greed, the seeds may grow into a full-blown malpractice suit. Not all untoward results culminate in litigation. Why? The "innocent" victim of a malpractice suit has usually broken one of the seven commandments of good doctor-patient relations:

1. Communicate with the patient and his family. Express concern, often more appreciated than your best therapy. And encourage patients to call if complications develop.

2. Avoid arguments with patients. Benjamin Rush (1745–1813), the distinguished American physician and political leader, wrote: "Make it a rule never to be angry at anything a sick man says or does to you. Sickness often adds to the natural irritability of the temper. We, therefore, bear the reproaches of our patients with meekness and silence."

3. Be wary of pressing for payment from patients in whom your therapy has yielded poor results. Threaten legal action and the disgruntled patient may respond with litigation.

4. Follow your difficult cases to resolution, arranging specialist consultation when indicated.

5. Don't be greedy. High fees, merciless dunning, and withholding care pending receipt of payment all tarnish the doctor's image.

6. Don't dabble in untried or experimental procedures. Stay within your depth, offering care for disorders within your training and experience.

7. Never, never criticize the patient's previous physician. You're only hearing half the story. What is the doctor's version? If the tale were truly told, the previous doctor's actions probably represented acceptable medical practice, but have become distorted by hate and anger. Sir William Jenner (1815–1898), the English pathological anatomist, observed: "Never believe what a patient tells you his doctor has said."

References and Suggestions for Further Reading

1. Bazelon L: Medical progress and the legal process. Pharos 32:34–40, 1969.
2. Chayet N L: Legal Implications of Emergency Care. New York, Appleton, 1968.
3. Curran W J: Medical malpractice in diagnosis. N Engl J Med 281: 312–313, 1969.
4. Curran W J: Tracy's Doctor as a Witness. Philadelphia, Saunders, 1965.
5. Gee D J: Lecture Notes on Forensic Medicine. Philadelphia, Davis, 1968.
6. Glaister J, Rentoul E: Medical Jurisprudence and Toxicology. Philadelphia, Davis, 1966.
7. Horsley J E: Testifying: How careless records can mess you up. Med Economics 48:99–111, 1971.
8. Kramer C: The Negligent Doctor: Medical Malpractice in and out of Hospitals and What Can Be Done About It. New York, Crown, 1968.
9. Long R H: The Physician and the Law. New York, Appleton, 1968.
10. Mann G T, Jordan T D: Personal Injury Problems Resulting from Trauma, with Special Reference to Automobile Accidents. Springfield, Ill, Thomas, 1963.

11. Medicolegal Forms with Legal Analysis. Chicago, American Medical Association, 1961.

12. Russell D H, Chayet N L: Law-medicine notes: Abortion laws and the physician. N Engl J Med 276:1250–1251, 1967.

13. Tozer F L, Kasik J E: The medical-legal aspects of adverse drug reactions. Clin Pharmacol Ther 8:637–646, 1967.

14. Watanabe T: Atlas of Legal Medicine. Philadelphia, Lippincott, 1968.

24

How To Survive
the Practice of Medicine

There is no creature in Scotland that works harder and is more poorly requited than the country doctor, unless perhaps it may be his horse. Yet the horse is, and indeed must be, hardy, active, and indefatigable, in spite of a rough coat and indifferent condition; and so you will often find in his master, under an unpromising and blunt exterior, professional skill and enthusiasm, intelligence, humanity, courage, and science.

Sir Walter Scott
(1771–1832)

From Attica to Athens, the lonely race is run. Disease threatens, and Death swings his broad scythe. But the runner dispatches them and speeds along his way, carrying the torch.

As it was in the time of Hippocrates and Aesculapius, so it is today. To survive the practice of medicine, the doctor needs strong shoulders to bear the burden of others' troubles, quick wits to avoid the pitfalls of practice, thick skin to withstand the rains of criticism, fortitude to act on lonely decisions, and humility to accept defeat, over and over.

THE CRUSH OF PATIENTS

The doctor with more responsibilities than stamina is often serving his own needs, not his patients'. Dedicated, but fatigued, he plods through the day. Accepting patients he lacks the time to treat effectively, he abandons preventive medicine, offering only "crisis" care. Incomplete examinations and rushed consultations crowd the day, and there is no room for the joy of medicine.

In the end, the devoted doctor becomes a leading candidate for the *JAMA*'s weekly obituary column—suicides and premature heart attacks, silent testimony to the folly of misplaced dedication.

Can this tragedy be avoided?

Yes, doctor, you can survive the practice of medicine. It takes only the soul-searching recognition of your limitations and a hard-nosed determination to respect them.

CAN A MEDICAL PRACTICE BE CONTROLLED?

It can and must. For centuries, successful physicians have governed their work load.

Specialization is the classic work-load regulator. Limiting his activities to orthopedics, gynecology, or psychiatry frees the doctor from the burdens of unrelated problems. "My practice is limited, you'd better call your family doctor or an internist about your abdominal pain."

The overworked specialist, swamped with cases within his domain, has another practice-limiting ploy. Accept only referrals. Appointments will be given only to patients specifically referred by another physician. This cuts the practice demands by reducing the number of callers, assures that another physician has screened out inappropriate cases, and allows the specialist to send the patient back to his referring physician when therapy is complete.

An age group limitation characterizes pediatrics, and other specialties have seen the light. The internist may shun children, and the pediatric subspecialties of cardiology, surgery, and psychiatry have afforded many physicians well-regulated, yet financially successful, practices.

Limiting the family practice is more difficult, often requiring ruthless pruning of problem offshoots. How about obstetrics? There's nothing like lingering labor to shatter the day's schedule. And a long night in the delivery room leads to a grouchy doctor the morning after.

Geographic limitations are important to doctors who make house calls. Doctors charge for their time, but few patients could afford the true value of a physician's time devoted to a house call 10 miles distant. Early in your practice, define your house-call area and decline to accept as patients those who live beyond. Ignore assurances, "Oh, Doctor, we'd never ask for a house call." Sooner or later, the unexpected arises, and the long-distance house calls begin.

Accepting as new patients only relatives of your present patients is another practice-limiting maneuver. In effect, the practice is closed. New patients are not accepted, but appointments will be given to parents, children, aunts, uncles, cousins, in-laws, brides, and bridegrooms of your present patients. The new arrivals will more than offset patients moving away, and most doctors are surprised at how rapidly a family-related practice grows.

The closed practice becomes a necessity in many areas. The average family physician can effectively care for about 3000 patients. With a large office and staff, the super-efficient physician can accommodate 5000 patients. Beyond that number, physician and patients alike suffer. Some "closed" practices quietly accept new patients one week each quarter or a month annually. Others accept relatives of present patients as they move into the area. Most busy clinicians find that if they accept only new arrivals in the household—newborn infants and newly married spouses—the practice will continue to grow.

Can a gargantuan practice be reduced? Béla Schick (1877–1967) compared the practice of medicine to heart muscle contraction: "It's *all or none.*" But when demand exceeds supply, the physician's efforts must be rationed by reducing the practice volume to somewhere in the Utopia between all and none.

A reduction in office hours is easier than you think. "Oh," you protest, "it could never work. I'd never be able to take Tuesday afternoons off." Try it. Pick an afternoon a week or two from now. Cross out the time in your appointment book and tell you aide, "I won't be seeing patients that afternoon." When the day comes, complete your consultations and leave. You'll see no patients that afternoon because none were scheduled. The reduction of office hours requires only the decision to take the step and the determination to see it through.

Odd jobs can balloon your practice responsibilities. When reducing a swollen practice, attack those time-consuming outside activities—school physical check-ups, employment examinations, and nursing-home coverage. Sitting on the bench at the football game each Saturday afternoon may bolster your ego, but if it becomes work, stop. And while paring time-consuming activities, eliminate the biggest hour-wasters of all—committee meetings. This includes service clubs and professional societies. Consider the last committee meeting you attended. Did the momentous decisions reached justify the value of the man-hours expended?

Some family physicians are finding that hospital care doesn't pay. If your office is located more than a few miles from the hospital or if you practice more preventive than crisis medicine, the hospital practice may include only a few patients daily, most of whom could be better treated by specialists during their hospital stay. And that small hospital population obligates the physician to service coverage responsibilities, committee meetings, and the daily journey to the hospital—weekends, holidays, and "days off."

Can you afford a hospital practice? Perhaps your life would be happier without it.

Will raising fees hold down or reduce your practice? Probably not. In fact, the reverse may occur. Americans demand the best, with price often the only criterion. The physician with the highest fees must be the best in town and may also become the most sought-after.

Is group practice the answer? It offers assured coverage and ready consultation. Better equipment can be afforded, and facilities don't lie idle during your time off. If you're a good organization man, go ahead. Most doctors aren't. Individualistic to a fault, the physician embracing group practice often finds the honeymoon ends abruptly with power struggles, rigid restrictions, and unsatisfactory doctor-patient relations. Yes, for many, the confinements of group practice are an exorbitant price for the tenuous advantages offered.

OFFICE HOURS ARE OVER

"Doctor, I know your office hours are over, but. . . ." Here's the threat to your survival, the welter of quasiurgent calls—babies with fevers, prescription refills, and hospital patients needing sedation at midnight. Your psyche can withstand a 10-hour office work day only if a silent telephone allows a few hours of evening relaxation.

Night calls are, of course, part of medical practice. The doctor's accessibility to his patients keeps the lines of communication open. Take your own night calls whenever possible, and when Johnny Smith's daytime office visit with a viral flu is followed by a 105.6° fever at 2 A.M., the call comes to you, not a strange physician lacking your familiarity with the case.

Trading calls with colleagues is a time-honored device, allowing short respites free of responsibility. Perhaps one full day weekly can be traded. The doctor who exchanges coverage regularly with another single physician soon finds he knows the patients of both practices, and his patients have the assurance of a second physician to call when emergencies arise.

Hospital residents are often employed to provide evening coverage for a busy practice. The resident gains valuable private-practice experience, and the doctor has his evenings free. But be careful. Choose your resident carefully. Don't ask a psychiatric resident to assume command of a busy general practice. Make sure his professional liability insurance includes the responsibilities he will assume. And keep open your lines of communication for consultation when difficult cases arise.

The answering service reduces the jangling of your home telephone. But beware the malpractice traps here. Curt replies engender patient hostility. Lost or garbled messages can lose your patients' confidence. Pity the poor operator, lacking your professional knowledge and experience, forced to deal with excited demanding patients calling for attention to symptoms that may portend disaster. Should she awaken the doctor or not? Will he bark at her for calling about a feverish child? Will the message wait until morning?

Once the answering service has accepted a call, the responsibility shifts to the physician. The operator is his employee, and the responsibility for her actions lies with him. A misinterpreted plea, a neglected symptom, and the doctor may be in trouble.

Automatic telephone answering devices are often used, particularly in small communities which, like mine, have no answering service. Perhaps this was a disguised blessing. My telephone answering device responds with a recorded message, changed whenever I am off duty. I begin by identifying the voice as a recording, alerting the patient that I am gone for a specified length of time, telling my anticipated time of return, detailing the coverage arrangements for the evening, and suggesting the next time office hours will be held. Reasoning that patients are reluctant to tell their symptoms to a tape recorder, I avoided purchasing the more expensive machines allowing callers to record messages. In almost all cases, the automatic answering device has worked well, at least as well as an answering service. And it's much less expensive. I receive no garbled messages. No irate patients complain of indifferent answering service operators. And, important from a legal viewpoint, the responsibility for securing medical attention shifts back to the patient. If you can count on your covering colleague and if the hospital emergency room will accept the occasional crisis when you both are busy, the telephone answering device may be for you.

Night office hours are anachronistic. Besides sapping your stamina, they can result in frequent evening interruptions on other nights of the week. Here's why. If you have evening office hours one night a week, patients will call on the other six nights inquiring, "Is tonight the night?" The answer? Work from sun-up to sun-down and use the evenings to restock your emotional and physical stores.

A second office in the home solves many problems, reducing night-time trips to open a darkened office or meet a patient at the hospital emergency room. Many patients with earaches, fevers, and minor lacerations can be effectively treated in your study at home. You will need a lightweight examination table, a suture set, splints, lidocaine (Xylocaine), syringes, and the diagnostic equipment in your black bag. Stock plenty of samples to treat patients until the pharmacy opens in the morning. The homemade incubator described in Chapter 13 keeps culture specimens warm, and perhaps your wife will donate a corner of the refrigerator to store culture plates, penicillin, and tetanus toxoid. Besides offering convenience, the home office allows a substantial income tax deduction.

Despite the best-laid plans of doctors, some annoying and unnecessary night telephone calls filter through. I'm going to pass on to you some words of advice offered me by a sage physician who had enjoyed 35 years of successful practice when I was preparing to greet my first private patients: "Doctor, when called out in the middle of the night to examine a patient with a trivial complaint, one that could well have waited until morning, and when you suspect you've been roused from your bed only for the patient's convenience, don't be angry. Don't harangue the family with your ire. Treat the patient to the best of your ability, smile, and *charge him!*"

GETTING AWAY FROM IT ALL

Vacations are important therapy for the doctor. Have you ever advised your patient with a nagging peptic ulcer to take a vacation, only to have him reply, "Doctor, when are you going to take your own advice?"

Your patients will survive without you for a while. Think about it. If your office weren't there, your thousands of patients would be receiving their medical care elsewhere, oblivious to your absence. And they can do so for a few weeks each year.

Frequent short vacations are often more refreshing than long ones. Last year I took a 2-week holiday. By the fifth day I was restless, and by the end of the second week, I was pacing the floor, itching to get back to work, and worrying about unanswered correspondence and unpaid bills. A 4-day weekend can recharge your batteries. A 1-week sojourn returns you refreshed, ready for action. Schedule your vacations at 2- to 4-month intervals, allowing you the happy anticipation of some leisure time if only you can survive the next few weeks.

Scheduling a vacation is as easy as eliminating an afternoon of office hours. Tell your secretary to draw a line through the page; then study the travel folders.

Need you go far? A surgeon friend told me once that his best vacation came when he turned his telephone over to a colleague for 3 days and remained home with his wife, enjoying his stereo system and an uninterrupted 72 hours.

Medical meetings offer endless vacation possibilities. Often held in exotic areas of equivocal scientific importance, the medical meeting vacation offers the twin advantages of congenial professional companions and an income tax deduction.

Let's sum it up. William Carlos Williams (1883–1963) observed: "It's the humdrum, day-in, day-out, everyday work that is the real satisfaction of the practice of medicine; the million and a half patients a man has seen on his daily visits over a forty-year period of weekdays and Sundays that make up his life."

The practice of medicine can be fun, and it should be. Plan your practice, recognizing your limitations. Learn the time-saving tricks of the trade, invest in the right equipment, and surround yourself with capable aides and colleagues. Plan time for relaxation and study. Charge reasonable fees, see that they are collected, and keep a watchful eye on your expenses. And, most important of all, afford your patients cheerfulness, respect, devotion, availability, and professional competence.

References and Suggestions for Further Reading

1. Brown J W, Robertson L S, Kosa J, Alpert J J: A study of general practice in Massachusetts. JAMA 216:301–306, 1971.
2. Craig A G, Pitts F N: Suicide by physicians. Dis Nerv Syst 29:763–772, 1968.
3. Ford A B: The Doctor's Perspective: Physicians View Their Patients and Practice. Cleveland, Western Reserve University Press, 1967.
4. Menke W G: Professional values in medical practice. N Engl J Med 280:930–936, 1969.
5. Olson S W: Medicine in the 1970's. Pharos 32:75–79, 1969.
6. Rashkis H A: Urban health services of the future. JAMA 217:803–805, 1971.
7. Rutstein D D: The Coming Revolution in Medicine. Cambridge, Mass, MIT Press, 1967.
8. Taylor R B: Limit your practice? Why not! Physician's Management 11:52–53, 1971.
9. Taylor R B: 1976: The year we lost our independence. Med Economics 48:189–197, 1971.

25

Launching a
New Medical Practice

How could a people which has a revolution once in four years, which has contrived the Bowie-knife and the revolver, which has chewed the juice out of all the superlatives in the language in Fourth of July orations, and so used up its epithets in the rhetoric of abuse that it takes two great quarto dictionaries to supply the demand; which insists on sending out yachts and horses and boys to out-sail, out-run, out-fight, and checkmate all the rest of creation; how could such a people be content with any but "heroic" practice?

Oliver Wendell Holmes
(1809–1894)
Medical Essays

Beginning a medical practice is like launching a new ship. The keel is laid with training. The hull, fore and aft, is joined with dedication and determination. The doctor treads the deck that is his office, and the white sails of his professional reputation flutter overhead.

Preparing to launch a new medical practice is a formidable undertaking, the new physician often unknown in the community, carrying a heavy cargo of debt, and not altogether sure that his ship won't founder and sink.

PREPARING FOR PRIVATE PRACTICE

The big day is coming, the culmination of years of training and sacrifice. By now the fledgling physician has already chosen his specialty, be it family practice, surgery, internal medicine, pediatrics, or one of the multitude of other specialties and subspecialties. But one more decision must be made. Should the physician entering the world of private practice join an existing group or open his own solo office?

The American physician, with a rich tradition of rugged individualism, has long chosen the solo route. Small offices, in urban, suburban, and rural areas, have characterized the medical "cottage industry."

During the past generation, a change has occurred. With increasing frequency, physicians have banded into groups. The West and Midwest are already group-dominated, and southern physicians are joining the trend. The Northeast, long the stronghold of Yankee independence, remains the domain of the solo practitioner.

At present, the winds of change are gathering force. The federal government encourages group practice by allowing loans at bargain rates. As the tidal wave of health maintenance organizations descends upon us, solo practitioners may find that medical groups are essential for survival. Certainly, group practice is the wave of the future.

During our generation, solo practice will remain viable, and the young physician's choice between group and solo practice should be guided by his temperament, rather than by a "rational" evaluation of apparent advantages and trends. More than any other professionals, physicians are mavericks. Some can be tamed, however; and if you enjoy the support of colleagues, planned vacations, and regular working hours, and if you don't mind submitting your will to the majority, then a group is for you.

A group is like a marriage—sharing assets and responsibilities. Each partner must pull his share of the load. Divergent philosophies, infighting, friction groups, and the inevitable shirker can sow the seeds of discontent. A smoothly functioning group is a happy union, but a discontented doctor can upset the balance with spats that may culminate in disillusion or litigation. There are few friendly divorces.

Some physicians should never join a group. The rugged individualist may cooperate with colleagues and consult freely, but bind him with rigid hours and shared income and he fights his reins like a wild stallion. Never happy until free, the strong-willed maverick physician will be satisfied only in his solo office. There he is free to make his own decisions

—set schedules, buy equipment, determine policy—and overwork to his heart's content.

The practice location will determine the character of the doctor's medical career. The area of the country, the community chosen, and the professional associates nearby will form the backdrop against which the drama of medical practice is played.

Recognizing the importance of delivering medical care to patients, young physicians are returning to rural villages, inner-city ghettos, and suburban communities that have long begged for medical care. Here is where the patients are. A solo office or small partnership can provide quality medical care whether located in a farming community or busy metropolis. In fact, the rural practitioner enjoys many advantages lost to his big-city colleague—personal esteem in the community, a knowledge of his patient as a person, and physical safety when making house calls. On the other hand, the city practitioner boasts availability of hospitals and specialist consultation, and the cultural advantages of metropolitan living.

The young doctor should choose a community to suit his personality and age. The physician who enjoys intellectual pursuits may be happiest in a college community, while the doctor who deals poorly with questioning intellectuals may find happiness in a farm or manufacturing community. The physician with cultural interests may be content only in a large city.

The far-sighted physician chooses a town on the way up. Many localities, particularly in the East and South, have reached their zenith and are experiencing an exodus of young people. These hardly offer golden opportunities for establishing a new medical practice. Other communities, blessed with unusual recreation facilities, access to highways, natural beauty, or expanding industry, are on the way up. These are ideal locations for the new physician. Young families moving into the area will welcome the new doctor in town.

Can the community support another doctor? Here's where the family physician has an edge. The general practitioner needs 3,000 patients to support his practice. With the shortage of family physicians in America today, it is a rare community that cannot support another family doctor.

The specialist must choose more carefully, particularly when limiting his practice to referred cases within his field. The pediatrician, internist, and otolaryngologist require a patient population of 15,000 to sustain a specialty referral practice, but the required number drops to 10,000 if the doctor is willing to perform general duties. The general surgeon, orthopedist, and urologist each requires a potential patient population of 15,000. The ophthalmologist seeking a specialty practice requires a community of 20,000 persons; if he is willing also to fit glasses, the requirement drops to 10,000 potential patients. The requirements for a psychiatric practice vary with the community; an urban population of 5,000 to 10,000 anxious executives and housewives will support a psychiatrist, while the same physician in a rural practice might require a community of 30,000 persons. The neurosurgeon and physicians in subspecialties should be wary of towns with a population of less than 30,000 residents.

The local hospital will form an integral part of the new practice, and before opening a new office, indeed before making a commitment to the community, the new physician should visit the hospital and discuss his potential practice with colleagues and the hospital administrator. Ask the hospital administrator about health care in the community. Is there a sufficient number of family physicians, or are specialists pressed into general practice? Or, are the specialties overloaded, and the under-worked family physicians competing for patients? Does the hospital administrator anticipate difficulty with an application for staff privileges? Will the doctor's access to beds or operating room privileges be restricted? What obligations are incurred by hospital staff membership?

Courtesy calls to potential colleagues are in order, including a frank discussion of the doctor's proposed practice. Do other community physicians make the doctor feel welcome? Indeed, is the feeling of welcome so overwhelming as to suggest that responsibility will be heaped upon the new physician? Or are the indigenous physicians cool to the likelihood of a competitor? Is hostility sensed? If so, find out why.

PLANNING THE NEW OFFICE

Should the new physician rent, buy, or build? Each has its advantages, and a careful decision is in order.

Renting a medical office offers the obvious advantages of conservation of capital and a limited need for planning. Rent payments are, of course, tax deductible. In an established commercial or medical center, parking is probably readily available and maintenance duties will be assumed by the management. The doctor must assure that the proposed rental office has enough space, avoiding shoehorning an expanding practice into cramped quarters. An existing medical complex offers the advantage of down-the-hall consultation. An existing office in a shopping center brings prospective new patients past the doctor's door, but as the practice grows, the blessing can become a liability as shoppers become drop-in visitors. A rental office suffers two major disadvantages:

There is no growth of equity in the property and the rental office has an air of impermanence. The doctor is what grandfather used to call a "renter."

Purchasing an existing office can offer advantages. A retiring physician may include his equipment and records in the bargain, greatly reducing the new physician's initial capital expenditure. The doctor buying an existing practice buys its reputation, good or indifferent. An existing office building has real property value, and the local bank should readily approve a mortgage application for a reasonable figure. The disadvantages? An existing office building may not suit the new doctor's practice. An older office may lack room for laboratory or x-ray facilities. The waiting room may be cramped, and the examination rooms may be inadequate. Is there room for expansion? Is adequate parking available? Is the neighborhood deteriorating, or are new families moving in? Will major renovations be needed, ballooning the doctor's investment beyond the building's potential resale value?

Building a new medical office is a formidable undertaking. The advantages are obvious—an office designed to suit the practice, with up-to-date facilities and ample elbow room. But perhaps the neophyte physician should forego this luxury for a few years. Even with bank financing, a considerable capital investment is involved, and the beginning physician will need funds for equipment and supplies. How many doctors leaving residency or the armed forces know what their private practice requirements will be? Might the underfinanced young physician build an undersized dream office? Might he, with limited knowledge of the community, locate in an unfavorable area? Certainly, ownership of his own office is a laudable goal for every physician, but its realization should follow several years of experience in practice and in the community.

EQUIPMENT AND SUPPLIES

The established physician probably gives little thought to equipment and supplies. Complacently, he places his weekly order and dispatches his monthly check to the supplier. But at any time, a well-equipped medical office probably contains $7,000 to $10,000 worth of equipment and another $2,000 to $4,000 worth of supplies. The new physician launching a medical practice needs these—all at once.

Office equipment and instruments are major capital expenses, subject to depreciation on federal income tax returns. Because the equipment chosen will be used for decades, economizing here may bring regrets later. The wise physician will search for quality, borrowing from a local bank to afford the best, rather than scrimping to his later sorrow.

The following is a suggested list of major equipment needed for a new general practice office:

X-ray unit, wall-mounted or portable
Electrocardiograph and accessories
Ultrasound unit
Diathermy machine
Ultraviolet lamp
Electrocautery unit
Microscope
Autoclave
Centrifuge
Laboratory system
Refrigerator
Incubator
Audiometer
Visual acuity charts
Cast saw
Adult scales
Children's scales
Wheelchair
Examination tables, one for each examination room
Operator's stools, one for each examination room
Examination room chairs, two for each room
Examination room desks, floor model or wall-mounted
Consultation room desk
Consultation room chairs
Adhesive-tape dispensers
Paper-cup dispensers
Paper-towel dispensers
Secretarial desk
Secretarial chair
Electric typewriter
Electric adding machine

Photocopy machine

Dictating equipment

Electric pencil sharpener

Open stack shelves for filing patient records

Filing cabinet

X-ray storage file

Electrocardiogram storage file

Chairs for waiting room

Pamphlet rack for waiting room

Bulletin board for waiting room

Children's play table and chairs for waiting room

Coat rack for waiting room

Umbrella stand for waiting room

Curtains for all windows

Waste receptacles for examination rooms, business office, and consultation room

The new office will need instruments. Some will have been collected during the doctor's years of training and others may be purchased from a retiring physician. Nevertheless, the new office should be fully stocked with first-rate equipment. Each examination room must have its full complement of diagnostic devices and instruments. The minutes and hours saved by having equipment handy will soon offset their original cost.

The following is a suggested list of equipment and instruments needed for a new general practice office:

Stainless-steel basins

Stainless-steel forceps holder

Stainless-steel instrument trays

Emesis basins

Urine specimen bottles

Binocular loupes, one for each examination room

Otoscope-ophthalmoscope sets, one for each examination room

Head mirror

Ocular tonometer

Suture sets, at least three, including needle holder, Adson forceps, hemostat, and sharp scissors

Ring cutter
Tourniquets, one for each examination room
Oral airway
Transfer forceps
Splinter forceps
Spud (to remove foreign bodies from the cornea)
Ear irrigation syringe
Bayonette forceps
Thermometers, oral and rectal
Sphygmomanometers, one for each examination room
Kelly clamp
Vaginal specula
Spoon curette
Cast spreader
Plaster shears
Stitch scissors
Thumb forceps without teeth
Bandage scissors, one for each examination room
Reflex hammers, one for each examination room
Stethoscope
Black bag for house calls
Portable oxygen unit
Urinary catheters
Nasogastric tubes
Finger splints
Magnet for removing metal foreign bodies from the eye
Nasal specula, one for each examination room
Urinometer

The initial stock of supplies must anticipate emergencies as well as allow the routine care of patients. As a rule, a physician in office practice orders supply stocks to last 6 months or more. Special consideration should be given to dated biologicals. Undated injectables and disposable products should be purchased in bulk to take advantage of lower prices.

The following list suggests supplies that might be needed for a new general practice office:

Gauze sponges
Tongue depressors
Professional towels
Disposable razors
Cotton-tipped applicators
Band-Aid strips
Elastic bandages
Casting plaster
Orthopedic stockinet
Cast padding rolls
Kling bandage
Vaseline gauze
Telfa pads
Adhesive tape
Bili-Labstix
Tincture of benzoin
Ethyl chloride
Acetone
Alcohol
Zephiran
Betadine
Microscope slides
Blood-agar culture plates
Tine tests
Disposable examination gloves
Disposable sterile surgical gloves
Disposable examination capes
Disposable syringes
Suture material
Xylocaine
Disposable scalpels and blades
Kleenex tissues
Paper towels
Paper cups
Walking heels for casts

Eye patches
Cotton balls
Disposable otoscope specula
Toilet tissue
Examination table paper
Electrocardiograph paper
Lubricating jelly
Adhesive remover
Distilled water
Pap smear fixative
Wooden splints
Butterfly closures
Tubular gauze
Disposable vaginal specula
Disposable anoscopes
Slings
Gelfoam sponges
Laboratory reagents
X-ray file folders
X-ray mailing folders
Alcohol prep pads
Sanitary pads
Disposable diapers
Air freshener
Topical anesthetic for the eye
All injectables needed for the practice

Stationery and forms will be needed. These should be ordered in sufficient quantity to last 1 year. All letterheads, professional cards, and business forms should be printed on top-quality paper. The cost difference between bond paper and lower quality stock is slight. Whenever possible, forms should be color-coded for easy identification. Many doctors have their forms printed to order by a local stationer; others order all office stationery and forms from the Colwell Company, 201 Kenyon Road, Champaign, Illinois, 61820. The following is a list of stationery and forms suggested for a new general practice office:

Letterheads and matching envelopes
Prescription blanks
Personalized note pads
Diet prescriptions
Certificate of professional care
School gym excuses
Receipts
Bill heads
Charge slips
Patient roster cards
Immunization records
Appointment slips
Request for medical record slips
Dunning notices for delinquent bills
Return appointment slips
Statement of office policy
Electrocardiograph reports
Referral slips
Laboratory request slips
Laboratory report forms
Manila mailing envelopes
Envelopes for dispensing medication
Blank medication labels
Audiograph report forms
Practice announcements
Face sheets for charts
Progress notes for charts
File folders
Other forms and instructions used by the doctor in his practice.

RECRUITING A STAFF

A congenial and efficient office staff can lighten the doctor's work load. Careful selection of employees is in order, and the doctor should not accept the first applicant who drops in. References should be demanded and checked. A telephone call to a former employer will yield a more candid response than a letter of inquiry. In general, the quality of a doctor's staff reflects his salary scale, and the physician paying a minimum wage will struggle with employees of minimal competence.

How does a doctor, new to the community, snare a bright efficient receptionist and dedicated well-trained registered nurse? A nearby nursing school or business college may be a good place to start. Recent graduates may be eager for experience in a doctor's office, and should offer enthusiasm and stamina. The new doctor in town may find Welcome Wagon a potential source of employees, as other newcomers enter the employment market. An employment agency may be helpful in large cities, since it usually offers the advantage of carefully screened applicants. Don't forget the value of word-of-mouth recommendations as your family meets young women in the community. If the word is circulated that the new doctor is looking for employees, applicants will soon arrive. As a last resort, an ad in the local newspaper will surely bring applicants, many with dubious qualifications. In most cases, the physician's name should be omitted from the newspaper ad and qualified applicants directed to a telephone number.

Few aides arrive trained for office work. The new secretary, fresh from business school, may be overwhelmed by medical jargon. A competent hospital nurse may be lost in the doctor's office, having never performed audiometry, determined visual acuity, or recorded an electrocardiogram. Training is in order, and hours spent here will pay dividends later. A list of standing orders for the doctor's aides is found in Chapter 21.

At least one full-time aide is essential to provide continuity. With one full-time assistant to hold the ship on course, part-time aides may be recruited from the ranks of women who would like to work but can't manage a 40-hour week. Several part-time employees can work alternate days during the week or one can work mornings and another afternoons every day. The use of part-time aides ensures that a trained replacement is always available when illness strikes, and vacation time doesn't leave the office staff decimated.

The physician's office should have a written personnel policy, detailing the relation between employer and employees. What does the doctor expect of his aides and what can they expect of him? Personnel policies will be as diverse as doctors' personalities, but each office should have one. The following is a suggested personnel policy for a solo office:

Probationary period:
> The first 2 months of employment are a probationary period, following which a decision will be made concerning continued employment.

Salaries:

All salaries are figured as an hourly wage and will be reviewed yearly. The usual work day is considered to be 8 hours. Overtime will be balanced by compensatory time off. Full-time employees are paid for the usual work week. Part-time employees are paid for the hours actually worked.

Sick time:

Full-time employees are allowed sick time as needed. However, after 2 weeks of consecutive absence due to illness, the employee is considered to be on leave without pay. An employee who will be absent due to illness is expected to arrange for a replacement or notify the doctor as early as possible. There is no provision for sick time for part-time employees.

Vacations:

Full-time employees are allowed 2 weeks paid vacation each year. After 5 years of employment, full-time employees are allowed 3 weeks vacation annually. Employees on vacation are expected to arrange for replacement during their absense. No vacation allowance is made for part-time employees.

Days off:

The office observes seven legal holidays. Part-time or full-time employees may take days off without pay as often as necessary, provided arrangements are made for a replacement.

Retirement fund:

After 3 years' service, full-time employees (those working more than 20 hours weekly) join the retirement plan (HR-10 Keogh Plan or Corporate Retirement Plan). Tax-sheltered contributions are made by the doctor (or corporation) at no expense to the employee. Employees working less than 20 hours weekly are not eligible for the retirement fund.

All personnel problems are to be discussed directly with the doctor.

JOINING THE COMMUNITY

Just as patients look to the physician in times of illness, the community turns to the doctor for judgment and guidance. The new physician can make his mark by joining community activities. Speaking at a PTA meeting or service club is a good way to get started. Certainly, a volunteer ambulance group would benefit from professional advice by a physician. How about advising a troop of Boy Scouts or Girl Scouts? The local Narcotics Guidance Council might benefit from professional guidance. Perhaps there is an opening on the advisory board of the Senior Citizens' Club.

Some physicians conduct health classes in the local school. Others provide a helping hand to prospective medical and nursing students. The new doctor in town, with more time than patients, might indulge his literary urges and submit an educational column to the local newspaper.

The young doctor's wife can advance his image in the community by participating in civic activities. Welcome Wagon is a good way to meet other newcomers in town. Citizens groups, such as the League of Women Voters, welcome new members. Other good entrees into the life of the community include church work, Parent-Teachers Associations, study groups, the American Association of University Women, college alumnae groups, theater ·groups, political action groups, and even bridge clubs.

Patients notice and appreciate when the doctor and his family participate in community life and are disdainful if the physician remains aloof.

As the practice opens, a brief dignified announcement in the local newspaper is in order. If in doubt as to the propriety or format, the new physician may ask the guidance of the local County Medical Society. The announcement of the opening of the new practice may be a paid insertion, following the format of the printed practice announcement. The doctor may submit a "press release," announcing the opening of the office; stating the street address, office hours, and specialty limitations; and describing the physician's medical training and qualifications. With the approval of the County Medical Society, a photograph may be enclosed with the press release.

Finally, the office has been painted, the carpet laid, the curtains hung, and the furnishings arranged. An open house may in order, with friends, relatives, and local dignitaries invited. Family and staff can serve refreshments, and the doctor can show off his new facilities, free of the pressure of a waiting room full of patients.

The next morning, the medical practice begins. The aides appear scrubbed and starched in new white uniforms. The doctor assumes an air of confidence, despite lingering doubts. After what seems an interminable wait, the telephone begins to ring and appointments are made. Soon the door opens and patients arrive.

Chart in hand, the nurse opens the door to the waiting room and calls an unfamiliar name. The new doctor in town is ready for his first private patient.

References and Suggestions for Further Reading

1. Aring C D: The distribution of physicians. JAMA 219:606–607, 1972.
2. Bogdonoff M D: Concern about patient care. Arch Intern Med 123:719–921, 1969.
3. Brignoli W H, Goering D D, Jones D, Kahn R M, Satell L, Longmire W T: The fee factor in patient care. Patient Care Volume VI 4:79–101, 1972.
4. Brown W J, Robertson L S, Kosa J, Alpert J J: A study of general practice in Massachusetts. JAMA 216:301–306, 1971.
5. Cotton H: Medical Practice Management. Oradell N J, Medical Economics, 1967.
6. Coulter D F, Llewellyn D J: The Practice of Family Medicine. Edinburgh, Livingstone, 1971.
7. Dimond G E: A safe physician. Arch Intern Med 129:129–130, 1972.
8. Fry J, Dillane J B: The general practitioner and his practice. Practitioner 190:-150–155, 1963.
9. Geyman J P: The Modern Family Doctor and Changing Medical Practice. New York, Appleton, 1971.
10. Geyman J, McNamara E W, Olian S D, Walthall W: Combined practice: How to find the right associate. Patient Care Volume VI 2:96–104, 1972.
11. Ginzberg E: Facts and fancies about medical care. Am J Public Health 59:785–794, 1969.
12. Kaplan N M: Community medicine as an academic discipline. Arch Intern Med 129:124–128, 1972.
13. Ragan C A Jr: Proposal: A ghetto medical corps in lieu of medical service. Res Staff Physician, June 1971, p. 82.
14. Rogers D E: Medicine will be better if we lead the change. Med World News 10:41, 1969.
15. Sheppard J D: The doctor's "business condition." Postgrad Med 47:202–207, 1970.
16. Stevens R: American Medicine and the Public Interest. New Haven, Yale University Press, 1971.
17. Susser M W, Watson W: Sociology in Medicine. New York, Oxford University Press, 1971.
18. Talbott J H: Biographical History of Medicine. New York, Grune & Stratton, 1970.

Epilogue: That the Knowledge Shall Not Die with the Man

Medicine is the oldest learned profession in the world and it is rooted in its past. Each successive generation of doctors stands, as it were, upon the shoulders of its predecessors, and the fair perspectives that are now opening before you are largely the creation of those who have gone before you. It is therefore reasonable to think that anyone who has spent a long professional life in medicine must have something to hand on—however small or modest.

F.M.R. Walshe
1952

Doctor, do you have a Laennec's stethoscope? Is there a clinical tip that you would like to pass on to the next generation of physicians? Or perhaps you have a unique scheduling system or collection procedure. How about the novel way you managed an injury last week, or removed a foreign body, or clinched a diagnosis?

I'd like to hear it. The history of medicine is being written now. Will you contribute?

Today I begin collecting for the next edition of the *Practical Art of Medicine.*

I need your help.

Robert B. Taylor, M.D.
66 Forest Glen Road
New Paltz, N.Y. 12561

Index

Page numbers in italic indicate illustrations.